Doris Humphrey:
The Collected Works
Vol. 2

DORIS HUMPHREY:

THE COLLECTED WORKS

Vol. 2

Air for the G String
Two Ecstatic Themes
Day on Earth

NEW YORK 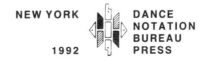 DANCE
NOTATION
BUREAU
1992 PRESS

Library of Congress Catalog Card Number: 78-67320
ISBN 0-932582-29-X (Volume 2)
ISBN 0-932582-28-1 (set)
Printed in the United States of America

Dance Notation Bureau, Inc.
31 West 21st Street
New York, NY 10010

Table of Contents

Acknowledgements

The "simple" task of assembling this historic volume has taken many years. It could not have been accomplished without the generous help of several colleagues.

We particularly wish to express our gratitude to:

Charles Woodford for his vision in allowing this publication to become a reality;

Jane Marriett and Muriel Topaz, notators, for their uncommon patience and expertise;

Ernestine Stodelle for all of her artistry and for the writing of the textual material;

Letitia Ide and Ruth Currier for their help in shaping ideas on characterization;

Lynne Allard and Letitia Coburn, autographers, for putting the notation into beautiful shape;

Tom Brown, Ray Cook, Virginia Doris, Els Grelinger, Jane Marriett and Lucy Venable, our extraordinary colleagues who contributed critical judgment by reading the notation;

Nancy Perry for her tenacity in getting this book well on its way;

Margot Lehman for editing the text and, with Alan Corneretto, for so graciously ushering the book through its final stages.

This book was made possible in part by a grant from the National Endowment for the Humanities, an independent federal agency.

* * * * * * *

This book is dedicated to Fredrika Blair, dance historian and writer, whose loving husband, Jerre Hastings, made publication possible as a tribute to her memory. This volume ensures that the work of a great choreographer will live on for everyone to enjoy and is a fitting memorial to a woman who had a great love of dance and its history.

The Dance Notation Bureau
1992

Introduction

If, in 1931, Doris Humphrey considered her solo, *Two Ecstatic Themes,* to be "the keynote to her mature work,"[1] then how shall we judge *Air for the G String,* created three-and-one-half years earlier? Shall we relegate the latter to the time when the young, impressionable choreographer was still composing within the folds of Denishawn and had yet to find her own language of movement?

By the same token, how shall we regard the 1947 *Day on Earth,* with its masterful use of archetypal characters? Dare we invalidate the artist's previous estimate of her own capabilities and declare *Day on Earth* — her eighty-fourth composition — to be the supreme example of Doris Humphrey's choreographic maturity?

Today, the comparative stature of these three works need not remain a matter of personal opinion or remembered impressions. Now defined as clearly as printed music or published text, the notated scores of *Air for the G String, Two Ecstatic Themes* and *Day on Earth* provide documentary proof of a talent that asserted itself at the beginning of a career and never lost its momentum. Here, in a single volume, is the concrete evidence of three fully realized conceptions, chamber-size works all, but each uniquely fulfilled within its own framework, be it quintet, solo or quartet. Lucidly recreating the movement within the contexts of bodily and musical phrasing, dynamic emphasis and visual design, these notated scores are ready for historical analysis and theatrical interpretation. The only missing elements are the specifics of each movement's motivation.

Would Doris Humphrey be disturbed by this last omission? Those of us who had the privilege of being directed by Doris Humphrey would immediately deny the need to analyze the meaning of each movement. Radical as this statement may seem to a viewer of Humphrey works, in which expressiveness is a dominant ingredient, the movement devised by this remarkable choreographer automatically discloses its meaning when performed correctly.

One has only to experience the smooth-stepping walk in *Air for the G String* to realize the calm it generates; or to raise one's hands slowly in the "prayerlike position" to be able to identify with the sustained notes of Bach's ethereal music. One has only to pull against the floor with the force required in an attempt to rise in the second section of *Two Ecstatic Themes* ("Pointed Ascent") to become aware of the emotional demands of such an exertion. And in *Day on Earth,* when the Mother reaches poignantly toward the just-departed child, the tale of a grief-stricken mother's motion becomes instantly clear.

In Doris Humphrey's vocabulary, the movement itself generated the emotional line, as well as being expressive of it. Her choreographic choices spoke for themselves. In studying these notated works it is essential that the dancer execute the movements exactly as choreographed — a double demand of fidelity on the part of the reader of the score and of the performer as interpreter. To ensure such fidelity, the services of an authorized coach, preferably one who has personal knowledge of the work, are required to supervise the reconstruction.

These considerations bring us back to the recognition of the relative choreographic stature of the three dances contained in Volume 2 of *Doris Humphrey: The Collected Works.*

The choreographic skill invested in *Air for the G String* is astonishingly mature for a choreographer who had only nine previous dances to her credit. Patterns merge one into the other without strain or interruption; the flowing forms created by the costumes, with their long trains and scarves, extend the vertical and horizontal lines of the movement upward and outward in perfect keeping with Bach's spiritually evocative *Air*. The dance emerges as a complete statement, visually and kinetically.

Two Ecstatic Themes, on the other hand, invades the personal realm. It suggests the premise that at the heart of feminine love lies the supreme paradox: a consuming desire to yield to the beloved unconditionally, and the equally consuming need to assert one's independence as an individual.

And *Day on Earth,* with its archetypal reading of human experience, contains the elements of classic drama. Only an artist in full command of her powers could unfold the ever-recurrent tale of man's journey through life with such simplicity and eloquence.

Who is to say which composition — *Air for the G String, Two Ecstatic Themes, Day on Earth* — is the more mature? Each in its own crystal-clear way is the product of a master of the art of choreography.

—Ernestine Stodelle

[1]Program, Repertory Theatre, Boston, MA, March 14-15, 1935.

Air for the G String

Choreography by
> Doris Humphrey (1931)

Taught by
> Ernestine Stodelle (1975)
> Revised (1980)

Music by
> Johann Sebastian Bach
> *Suite No. 3 in D Major,* "Air"

Notation by
> Jane Marriett (1975)
> Revised (1980)

Premiere: Doris Humphrey and Charles Weidman and students of the Denishawn School, Little Theatre, Brooklyn, New York, March 24, 1928.

Notated version: as taught by Ernestine Stodelle to the José Limón Dance Company, Manhattanville College, Purchase, New York, July, 1975. First performed July 19, 1975.

Running Time: 4:45 minutes.

Score Checked by: Ray Cook, Els Grelinger and Lucy Venable.

Autography by: Lynne Allard.

This score was made possible, in part, with the public funds from the New York State Council on the Arts, the National Endowment for the Arts and the members of the Dance Notation Bureau.

This seal signifies that the notation contained in this work has been approved and meets the qualifications for a Labanotation score as set forth by the Dance Notation Bureau.

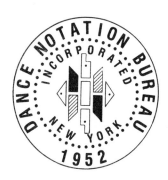

Historical Background

Viewed today, Doris Humphrey's serenely flowing *Air for the G String* might well appear anachronistic. Its peaceful configurations have little or nothing to do with the complex, breathless intensities of contemporary life. Suggestively Renaissance in costuming, with its long golden scarves and pastel sheath-like dresses recalling the saintly figures of a Fra Angelico painting, the dance seems far removed from the secular feverishness of the late twentieth century.

Nor does *Air for the G String* belong to the year of its birth — 1928 — when western civilization was still cracking under the penalties of World War I. Dreamily evocative of a realm outside the pale of ordinary existence, this cloudless quintet states its theme with the unhurried calm of a classic gesture.

Yet, with each viewing, the composition's pure, smoothly evolving forms become more meaningful to a dance public that has been increasingly exposed to the blandishments of technical virtuosity. Showmanship may dazzle, but when its fireworks leave no significant afterglow, the mind remains unnourished and still seeks aesthetic gratifications. It would seem that from the very outset of her career as an independent choreographer, Doris Humphrey was concerned with the imperishable beauty of simple, unpretentious movement.

Not one motion is exhibitionistic or self-projecting. Not one dancer stands out soloistically. Even Doris Humphrey in her rendering of the central role — a role she assumed for the first and only time in the 1934 film[1] — blends into the overall design, which has the quality of a spiritual ritual. Drawn together by an innerly felt communion with each other and with the noble, ecclesiastical tones of Johann Sebastian Bach's *Air* (from his Third Orchestral Suite), their relationship is one of luminous accord.

As the ritual commences, the five women are silhouetted in a cluster downstage, their backs to the audience, their voluminous silk scarves heaped in soft, pillow-like mounds on the stage's edge behind them. With the music's first measure, they move slowly upstage, lifting their hands before like votive offerings and opening their arms in a widespread gesture. At the crest of this movement, the central figure turns toward the audience with upraised arms. Simultaneously, the others face front, and after soft, gracious motions toward one another, they gradually form a circle stage center.

Thus begins Doris Humphrey's first choreographic evocation of her belief in "the nobility that the human spirit is capable of...,"[2] a theme she used ten years later when stirred by the magnificent sonorities of Bach's *Passacaglia and Fugue in C Minor.*

The clue to Humphrey's creative response to Bach's *Air* can be found in her foreword to the posthumously published *The Art of Making Dances.* She states, "... when I was a very small child... I heard Bach's *Air for the G String,* which so struck me to the heart that it was almost the first dance I composed as an independent choreographer." And she adds, "So music was my first love and I was led to dance through that."[3]

Note that Bach's music is referred to as *Air for the G String*, a prepositional variation (possibly Humphrey's unwittingly) of *Air on the G String*, the title of a popular nineteenth-century version of Bach's piece arranged by the German violinist August Wilhelmj in which the aria is played entirely on the G string of the violin, a virtuosic manipulation of fingering in those days.[4] What is important, however, is that Doris Humphrey's response to Bach's *Air* resided within her for well over two decades until she found, at the age of thirty-four, not only the movement to express her feelings, but also the form in which she could present them. Still retaining the title of her first impression, Doris Humphrey premiered *Air for the G String* on March 24, 1928, at the Little Theatre in Brooklyn.

Clearly, in this period of her choreographic development Doris Humphrey was concerned with the nonliteral translation of aural tonalities and rhythms into the physical dynamics of an independently created dance structure. *Air for the G String* was no mere conversion of musical motifs into kinetic action, but a choreographic entity that reflected the spirit of Bach's rich harmonies without mirroring the music's recurring themes.

While the dancers do not soar with the aria's climbing cadences but are tranquilly grounded in the smoothest of walking steps, the rise and fall of their cowl-draped scarves maintain the music's lofty mood. Choreographic patterns unfold with striking clarity. At one moment, the four dancers surround the central figure as she slips into their midst with an upward-swirling spiral. But almost immediately, the circle dissolves, and within a single measure the dancers have formed a stage-wide line and are advancing toward the audience, arms outstretched as the music swells. Then, almost imperceptibly the line divides into two asymmetrical groupings. Only at the end is there a held position, but not for long. With the ritard of the final chord, the lights fade, and the audience is left with a vision as elusive as a dream.

Spiritually akin to Bach's transcendent *Air,* Doris Humphrey's *Air for the G String* stands beyond the touch of time. — *E.S.*

Movement Analysis

Dance form is logical, but it is all in the realm of feeling, sensitivity and imagination... [5]

Paramount among the movement qualities that infuse *Air for the G String* with a special radiance is that of *sustained flow*. It is best seen in the quiet, even-paced walk that coincides with the underlying beat of Bach's long melodic cadences. Each step carries the body forward with a sense of wholeness. The leg is extended without hesitancy or stiffness. The arched, softly pointed foot carries the weight smoothly and confidently as the dancer advances toward some clearly felt goal.

Another movement quality is that of *harmoniousness*. The gentle legato gestures convey a fullness of feeling that is communicated from one dancer to the other, as, for example, in the unison sideways walk to the left (phrase 1, measures 9-12) in which each member of the ensemble looks backward toward the dancer on her right. The lean of the body assumes a firm, but softly gracious curve.

First evident in the opening movement of the dance — and repeated elsewhere — is a prayerlike position of the hands. The slightest pressure is required: thumb alongside of thumb with the other fingers reaching foward and upward without tension.

The backward slant of the body in the procession that leads upstage (phrase 3, measures 9-12) becomes decidedly oblique as the dancers begin to move in profile to the audience. Called in modern dance vernacular "the hinge position," the oblique tilt is created by a forward lift of the hips causing the weight of the torso to be borne chiefly by the femur quadriceps. A feeling of breath-filled suspension lifts the upper body as the hands gradually release their prayerlike position and fall alongside the hips.

The use of the breath serves as the fundamental impulse behind the rise and fall of the phrased movements. The most evident examples of such phrasing are "the billows" (phrase 6, measures 1-4), which are created when two and then three of the dancers sweep their arms backward and immediately upward before advancing alternately into a concentrically closing circle. The backward successional motion scoops the scarves upward, filling them with air; as the dancers step toward each other with hands pressed forward and downward, the airborne scarves subside. Performed in counterpoint as a group, the billows section has the looping effect of wave-like movements that build to a harmonious climax with all five dancers forming a closely knit circle with intertwined arms (phrase 6, measure 8).

Only repeated rehearsing with the scarves will bring about the necessary relaxed feeling for judging distances that must be observed between the dancers. Certain group formations, however, will always present hazards as far as the dangers of stepping on one another's scarves are concerned: notably, the confined circle (phrase 4, measures 5-8) when the central figure slips into the middle of the group. She must avoid stepping on any of the trains that are curled up on the floor due to the preceding configuration (phrase 4, measures 1-4). Once she is in the center, the two sets of dancers that flank her should be free to step backward unencumbered before proceeding forward with her in the wide line that brings the group downstage in unison.

The concluding movements of the dance (phrase 6, measures 9-12) are similarly complicated. To take lateral positions across the stage for the final gesture, the four dancers have to file past one another, stepping across each other's trains in advance of the central figure's walk upstage. The eyes should be focused forward not downward, and the illumination in the face, which should have been evident in varying expressions throughout the entire dance, now conveys an ultimate sense of consecration.

The last measure of the music finds the central figure midstage with her arms slowly extending sideways, while her acolytes — two on each side — after reaching toward her reverently turn away in profile with their hands stretched before them in the prayer position as the lights dim. — *E.S.*

[1] The recreation of *Air for the G String* was made possible through the study of the 1934 film.

[2] Doris Humphrey, Letter to John Martin, 1943.

[3] Doris Humphrey, *The Art of Making Dances* (New York: Rinehart & Company, Inc., 1959), p. 9.

[4] For the information regarding the nineteenth-century version of Bach's original title, the author is indebted to Neil Ross.

[5] Doris Humphrey, *The Art of Making Dances,* p. 31.

Resultant Scarf Positions

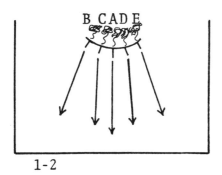

1-2

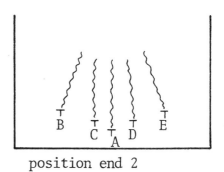

position end 2

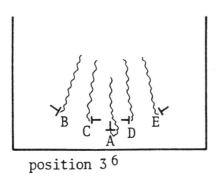

position 3 ^{6}

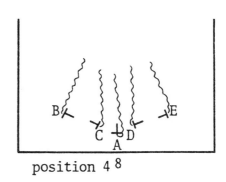

position 4 ^{8}

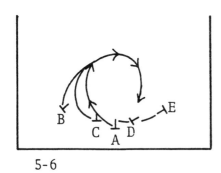

5-6

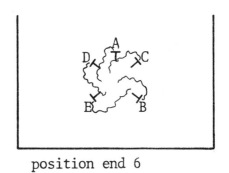

position end 6

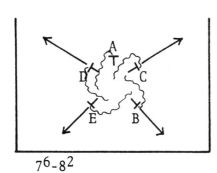

7^6-8^2

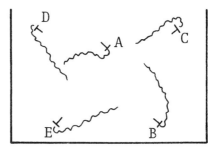

position end 8

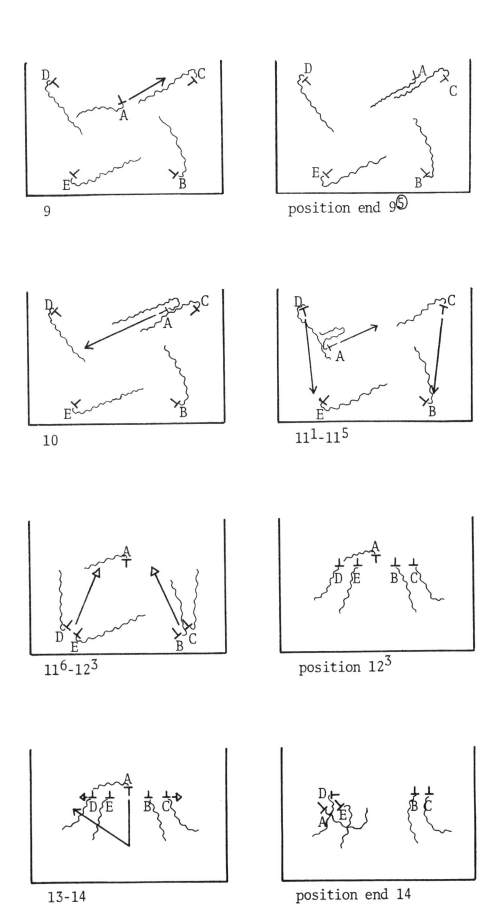

9

position end 9⑤

10

11¹-11⁵

11⁶-12³

position 12³

13-14

position end 14

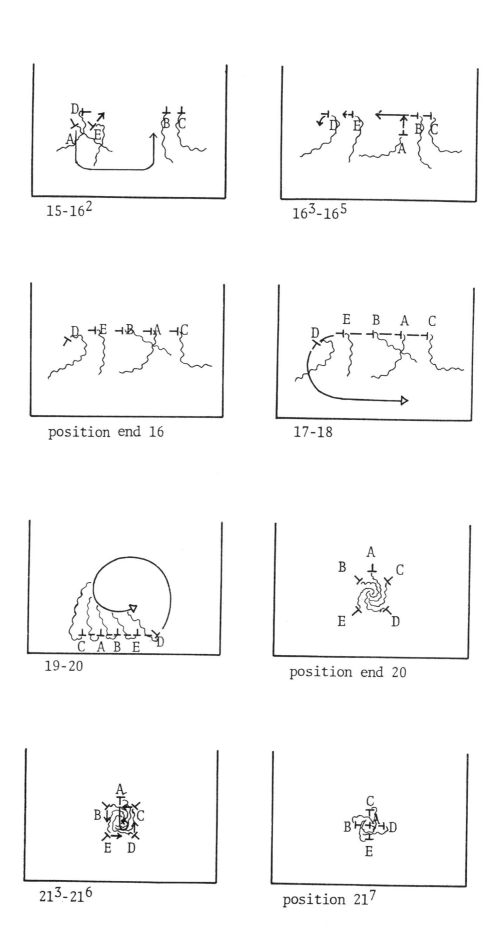

15-16²

16³-16⁵

position end 16

17-18

19-20

position end 20

21³-21⁶

position 21⁷

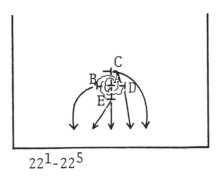

22^1-22^5

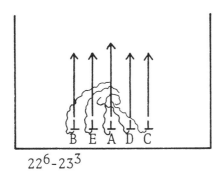

22^6-23^3

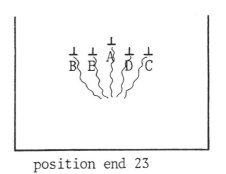

position end 23

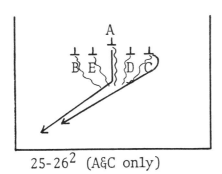

25-26^2 (A&C only)

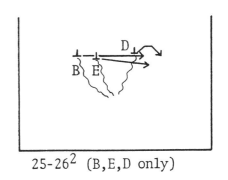

25-26^2 (B,E,D only)

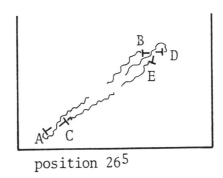

position 26^5

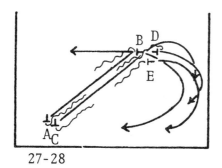

27-28

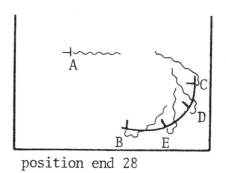

position end 28

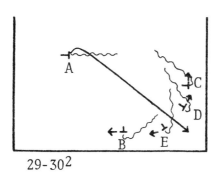

29-30^2

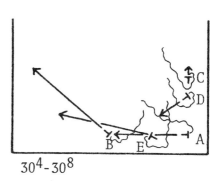

30^4-30^8

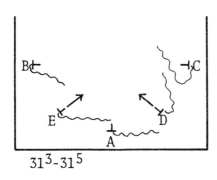

31^3-31^5

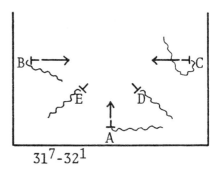

31^7-32^1

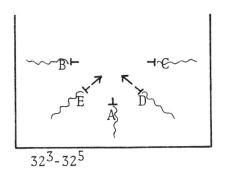

32^3-32^5

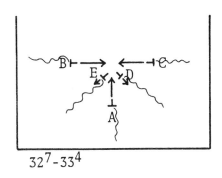

32^7-33^4

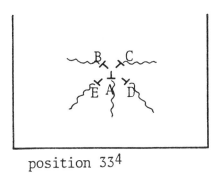

position 33^4

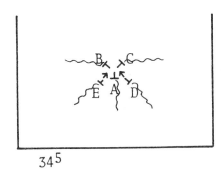

34^5

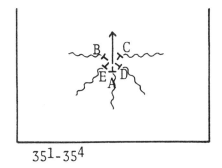

35^1-35^4

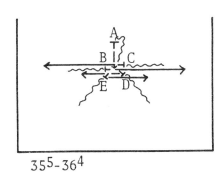

35^5-36^4

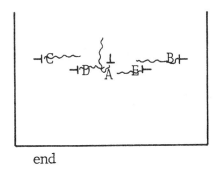

end

Glossary

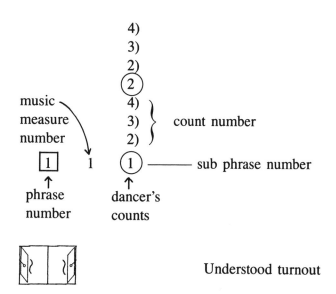

music measure number → 1

phrase number ↑

dancer's counts ↑

count number

sub phrase number

Understood turnout

The torso is often held slightly back so that the "scarf" will not catch.

The foot is understood to point on leg gestures, or a "Doris foot" may be used instead: .

Hands are always soft.

Movement breath, whole body rises slightly with inhalation accompany movement (see p. 18 m. 2). An might also the

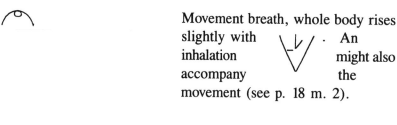

Steps have a gliding quality .

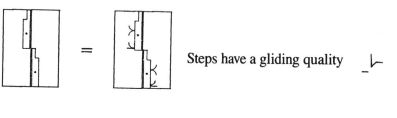

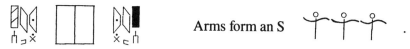

Arms form an S .

Hold from the standard system of reference.

(See A p. 20 m. 3 - The arms stay side middle from the standard system of reference.)

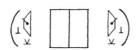

You look at the person, but the whole front surface of the head need not point directly at them. (See p. 22)

Path deviations are probably bigger than written. The exact size is left to the interpretation of the performer. (See A p. 20 m. 3)

Undeviating path, front judged from after the turn is completed. (See A p. 30 m. 14 - arms will end side middle)

Design Drawing - The body part indicated draws the design indicated within the path sign, starting at the dot. The design is drawn as if it lay on the surface indicated. (See 1979 ICKL papers)

For example see p. 30:

The design is situated horizontally below the free end of the arm. The arm draws the design beginning at the dot.

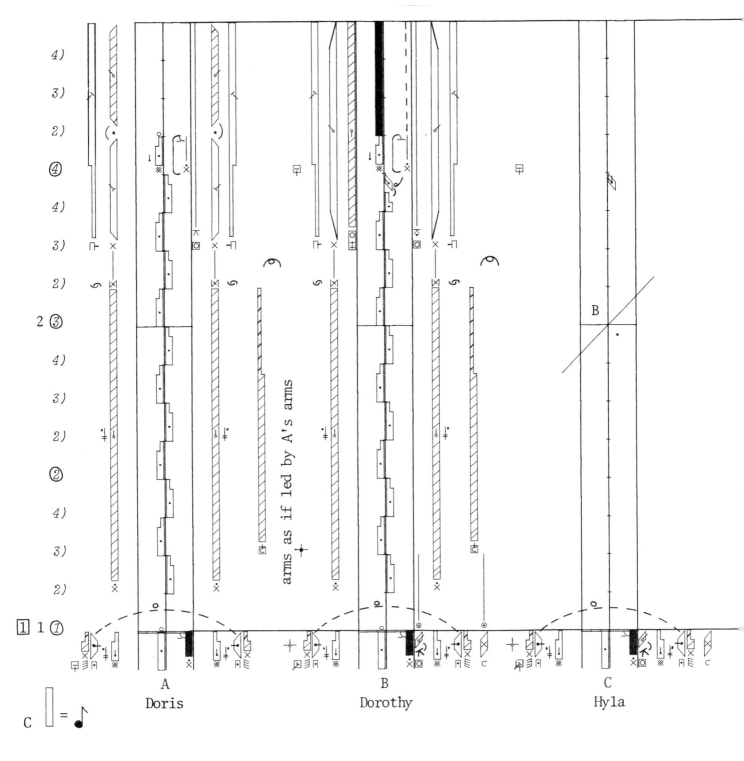

A
Doris

B
Dorothy

C
Hyla

arms as if led by A's arms

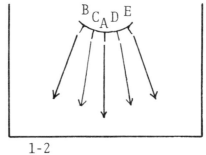

1-2

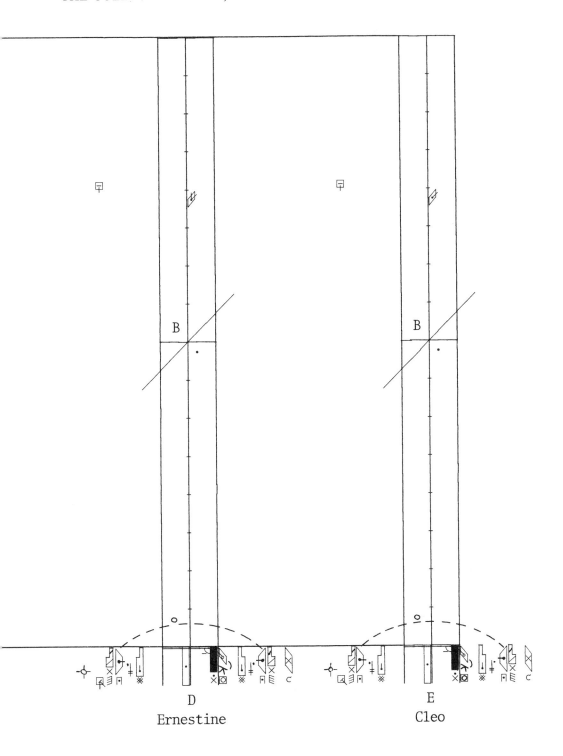

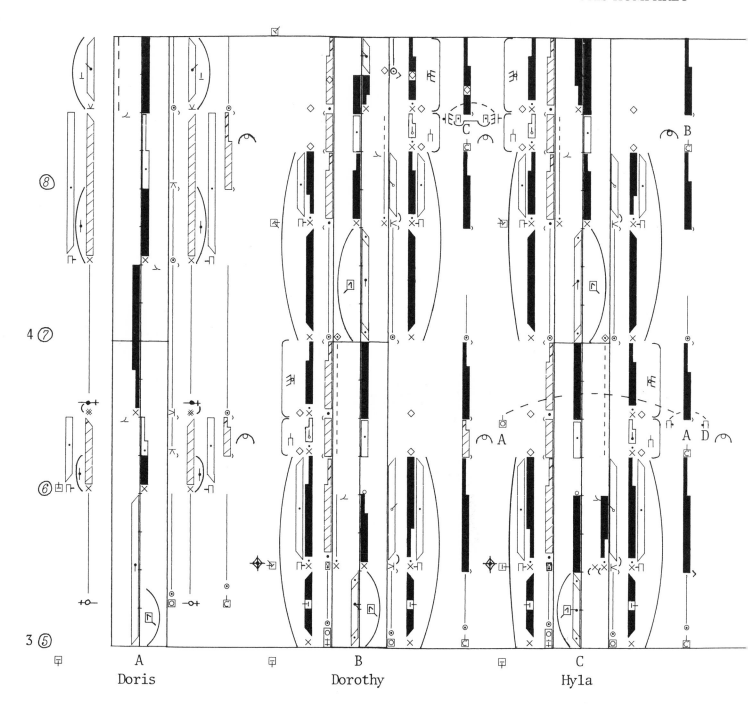

A
Doris

B
Dorothy

C
Hyla

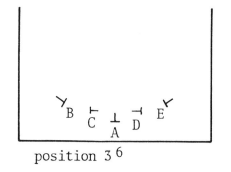

position 3 6

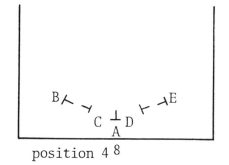

position 4 8

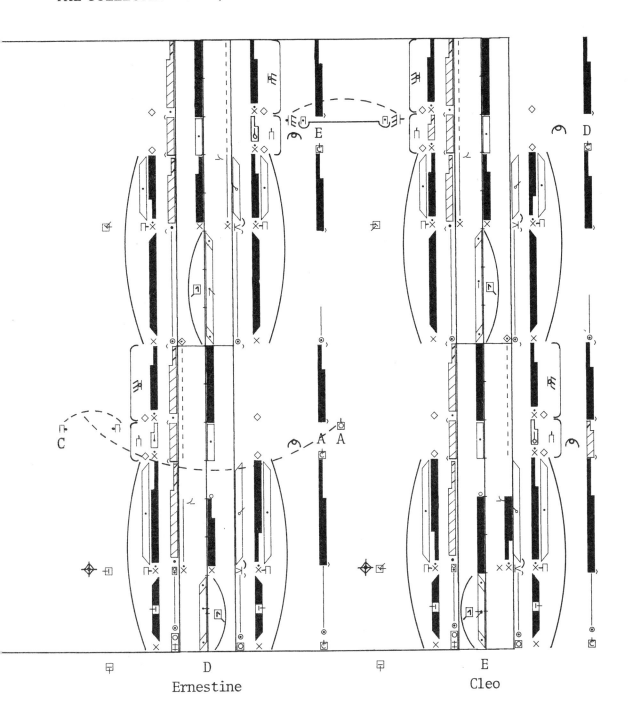

Ernestine

Cleo

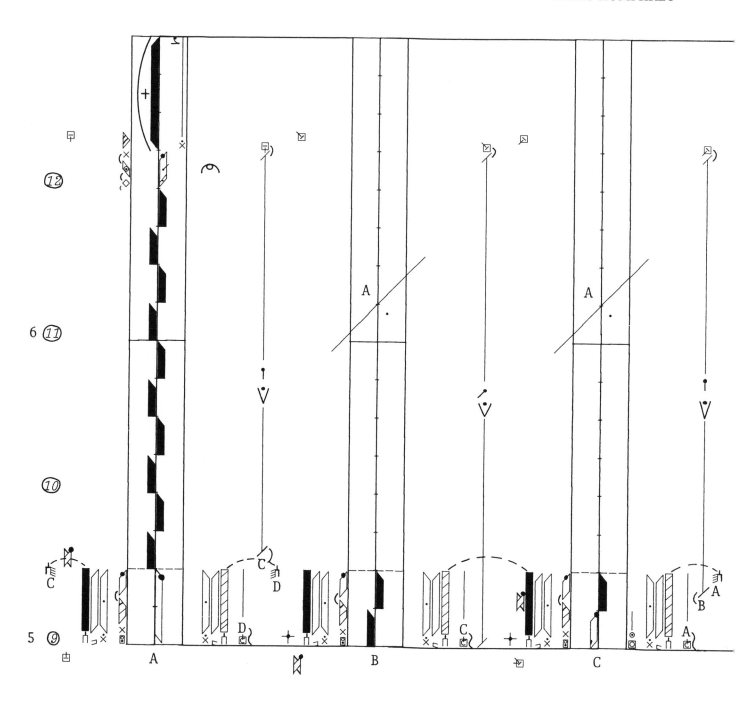

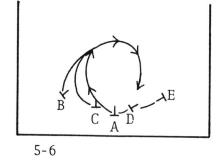

5-6

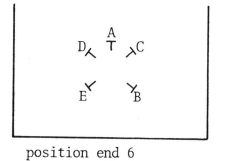

position end 6

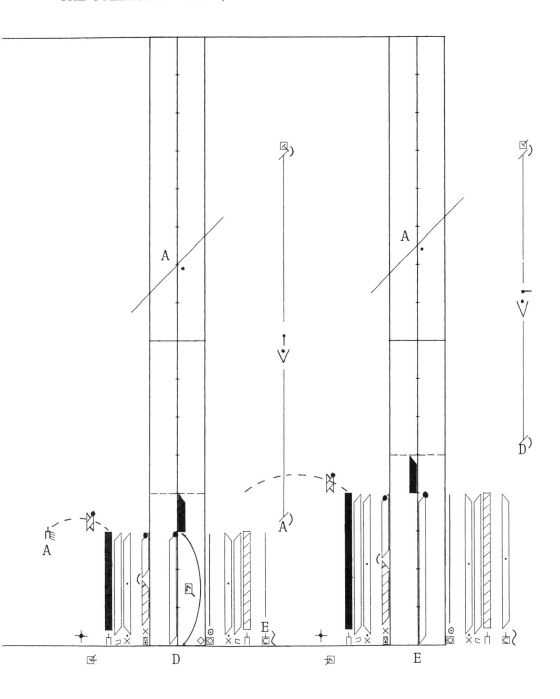

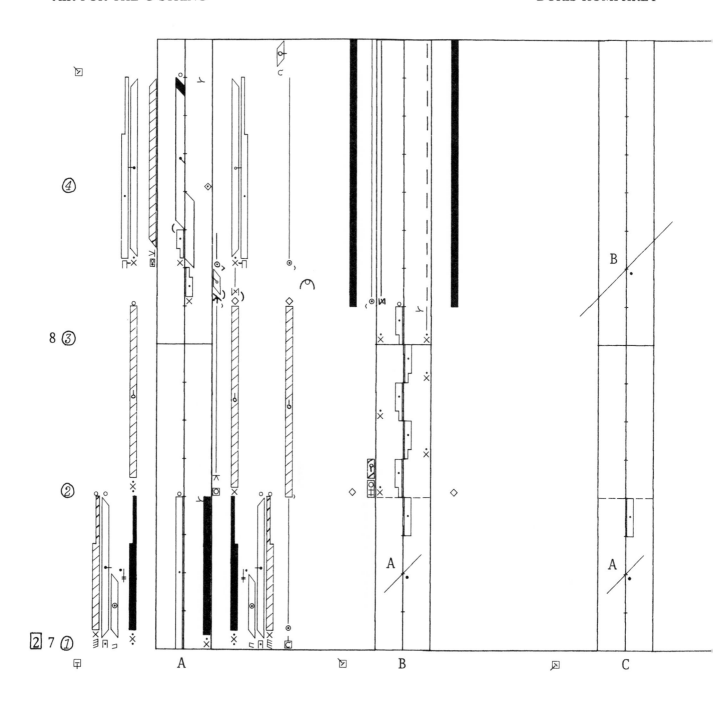

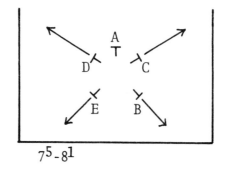

$7^5\text{-}8^1$

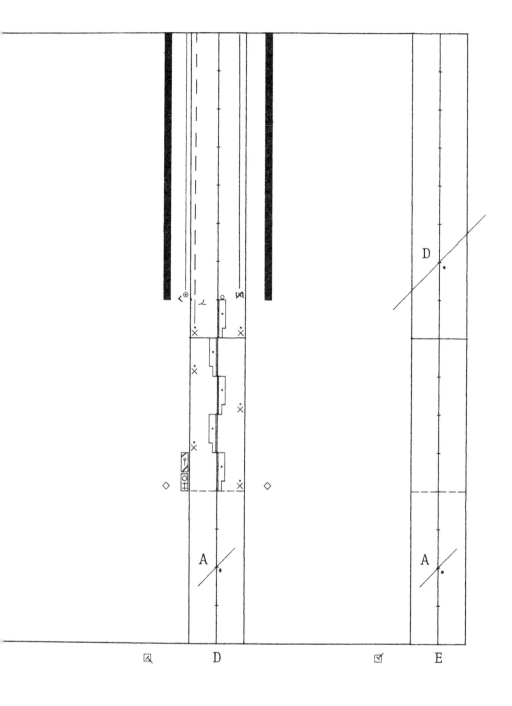

M. 95–97
movement passes from
through the body
and out the E

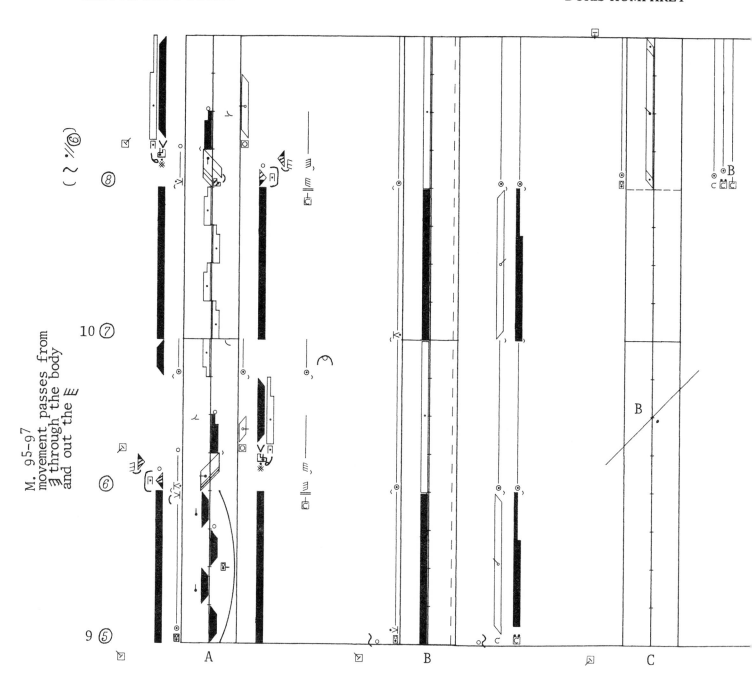

A B C

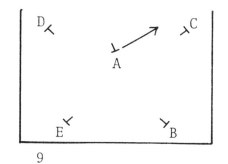

9

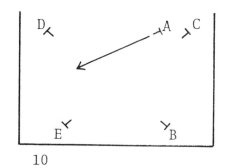

10

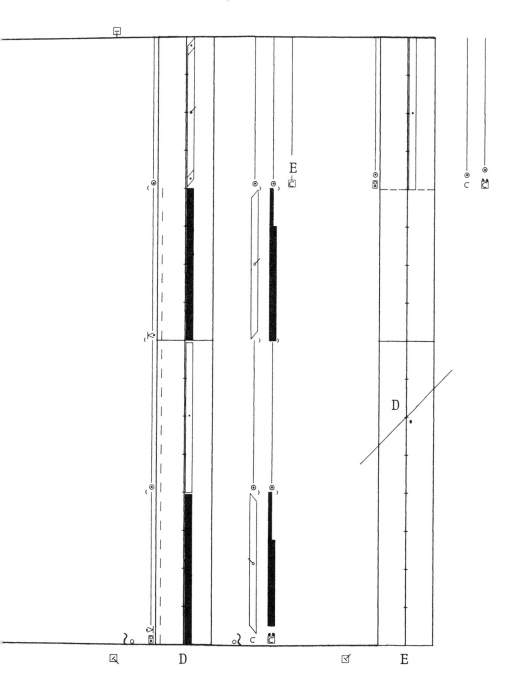

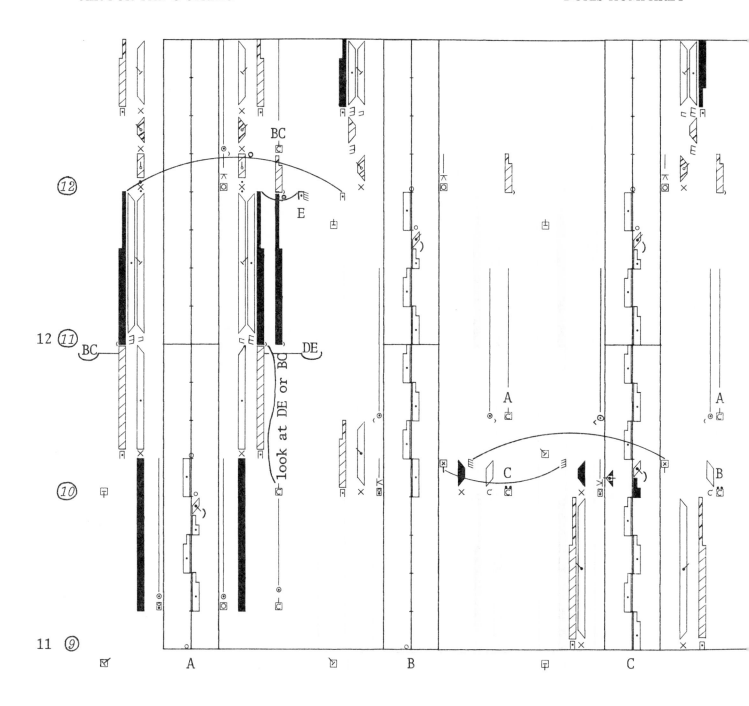

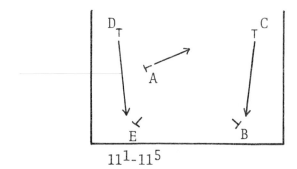

11^1-11^5

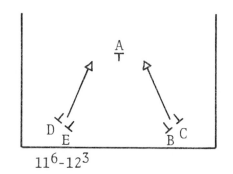

11^6-12^3

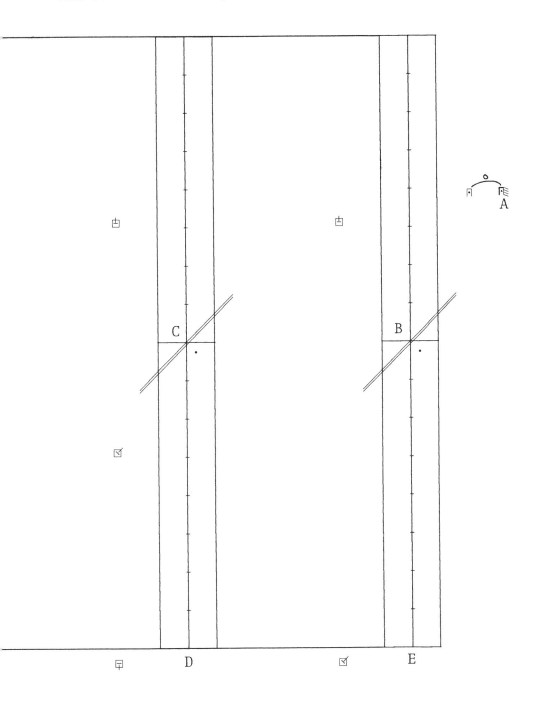

position 12^3

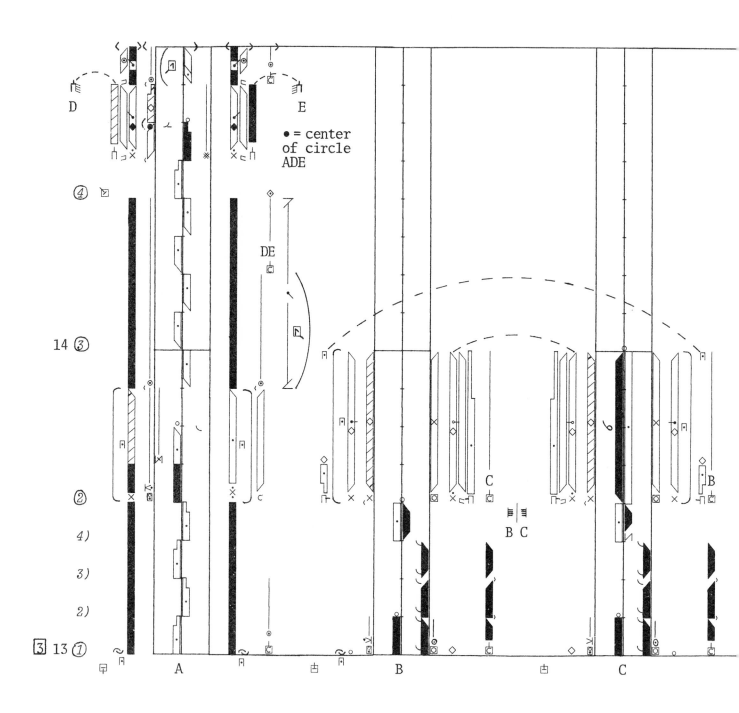

● = center
of circle
ADE

DE

14-14

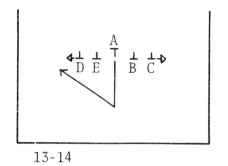

position end 14

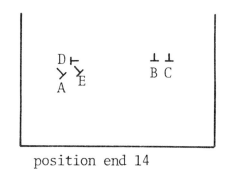

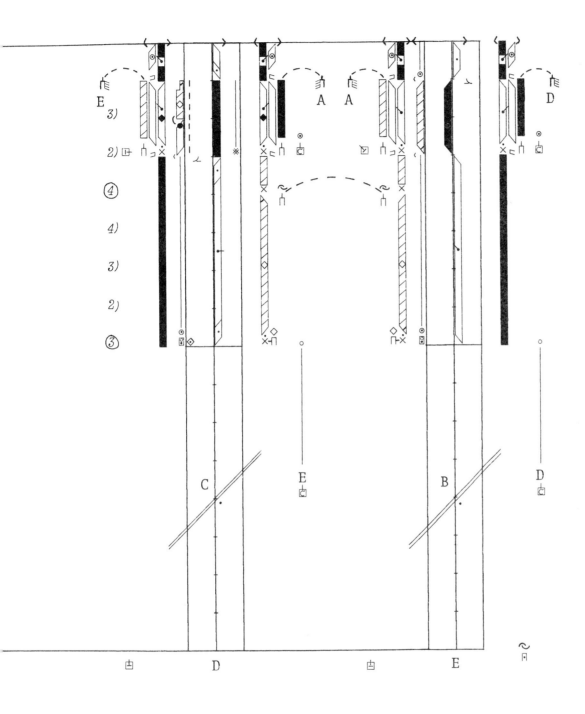

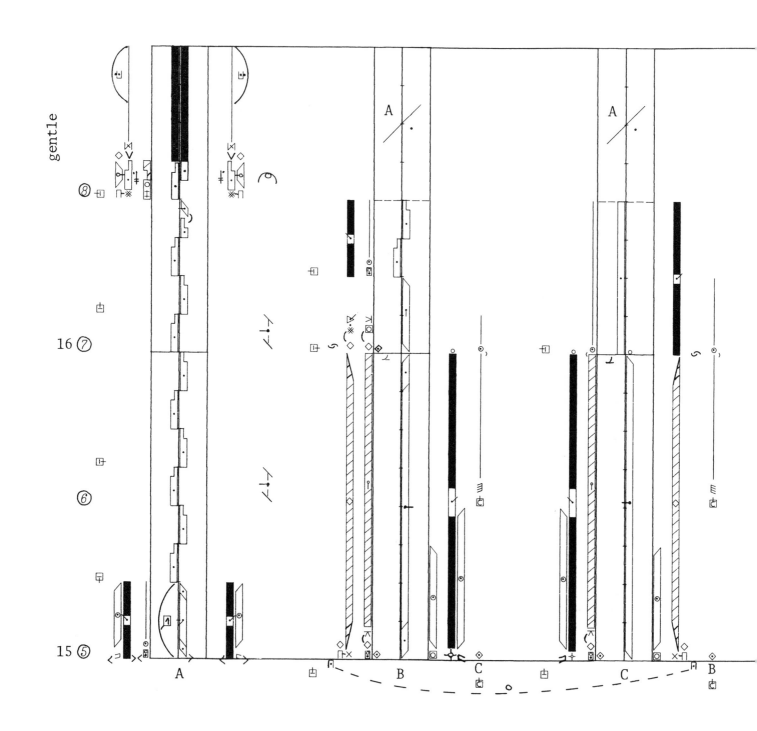

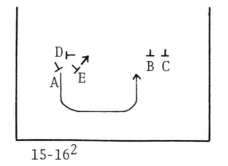

15-16²

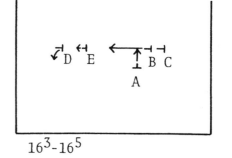

16³-16⁵

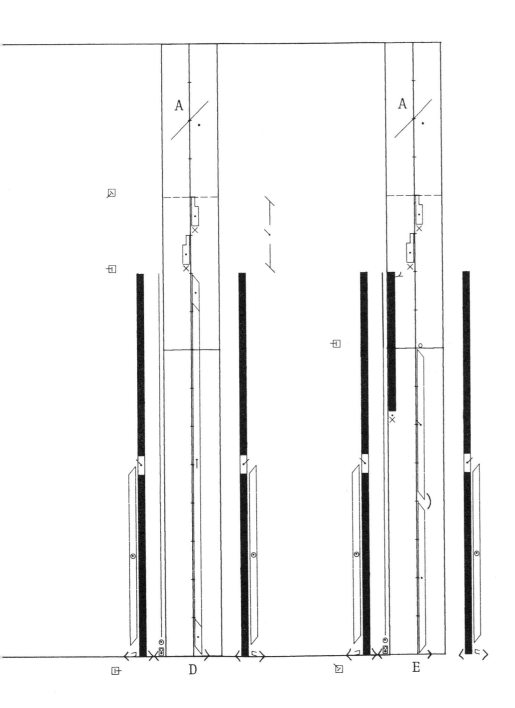

position end 16

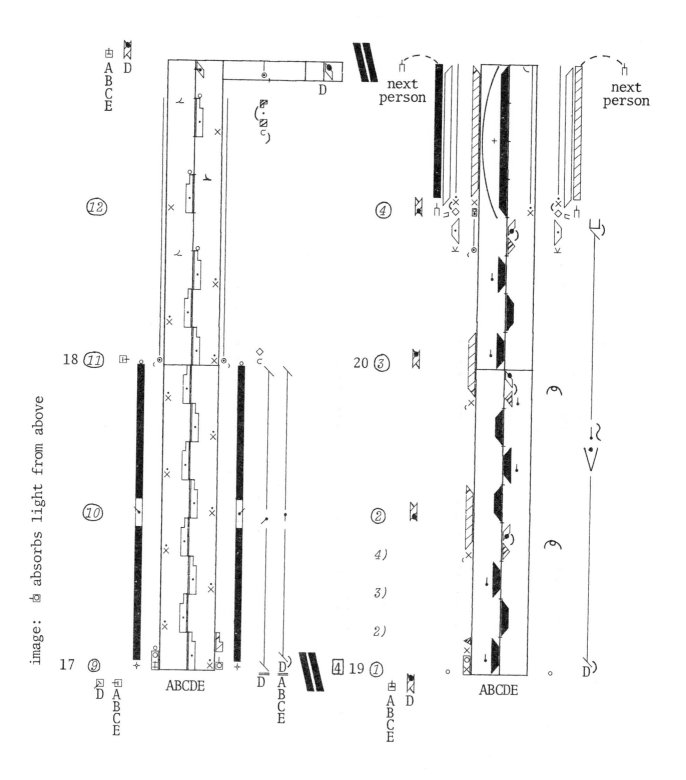

image: ☐ absorbs light from above

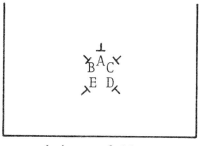

position end 20

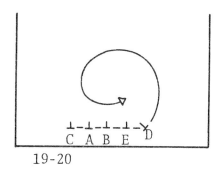

19-20

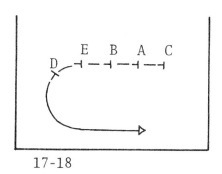

17-18

step over scarf

slide scarf
with feet

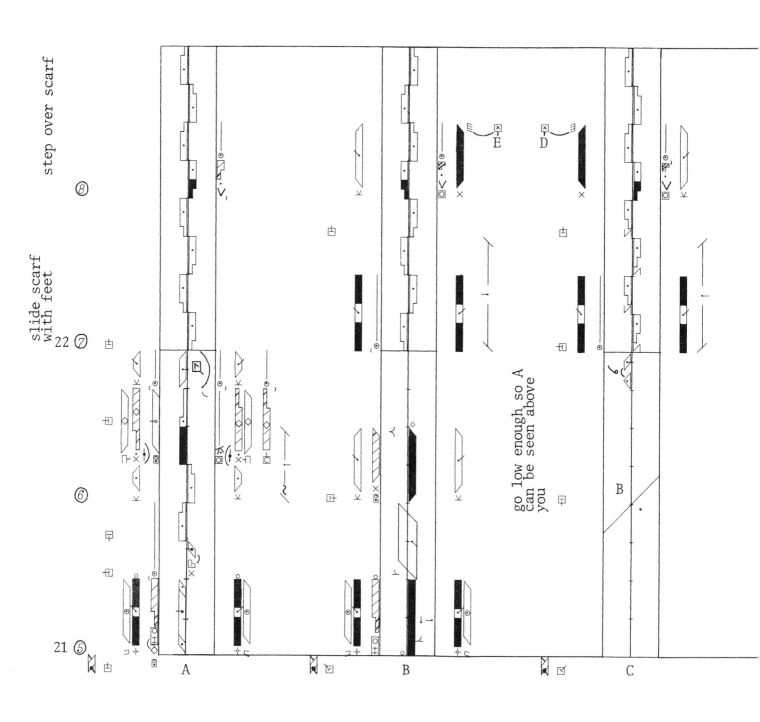

go low enough so A
can be seen above
you

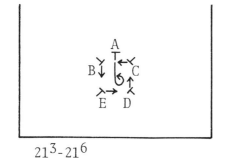

21³-21⁶

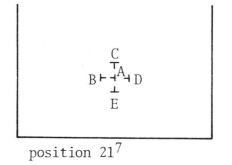

position 21⁷

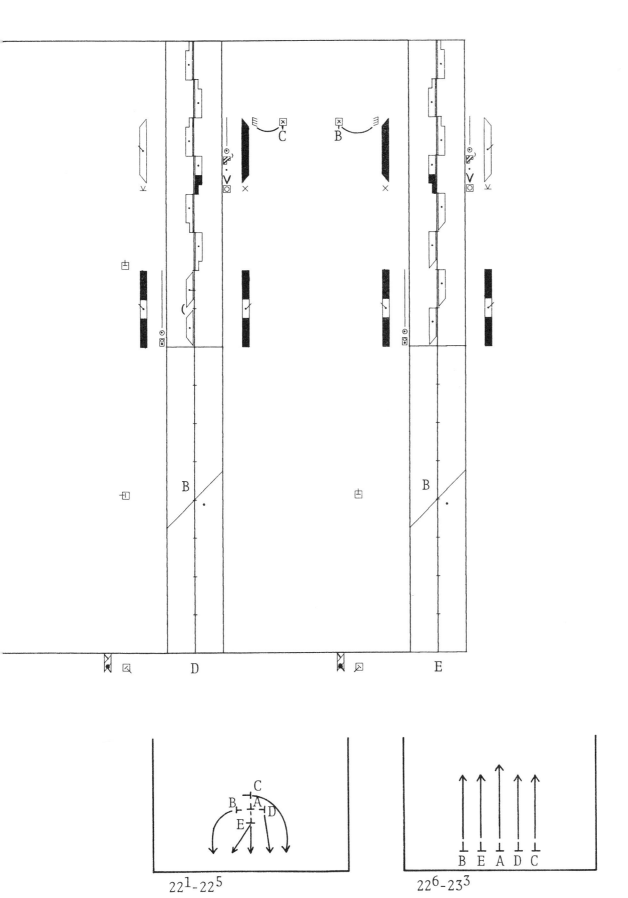

22^1-22^5

22^6-23^3

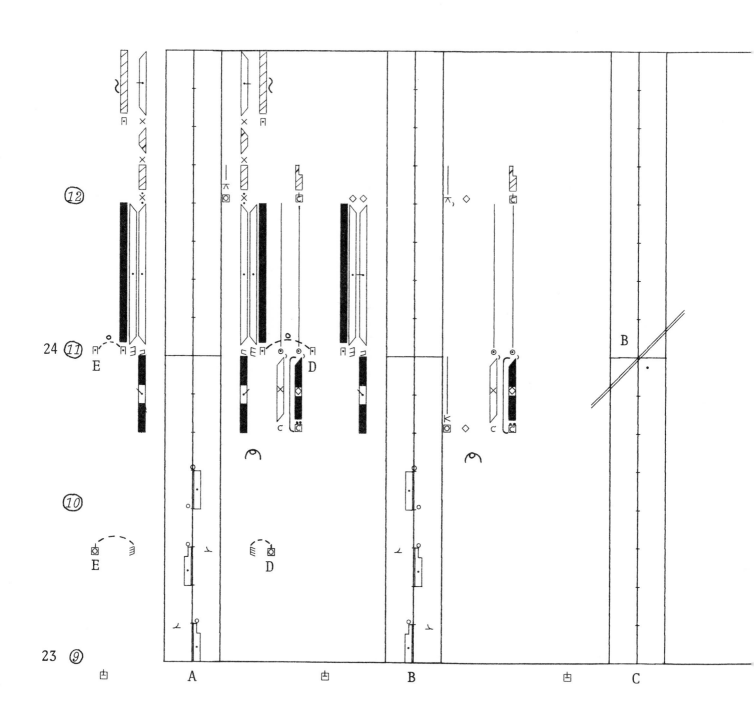

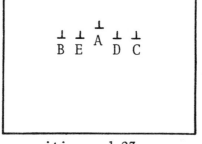

position end 23

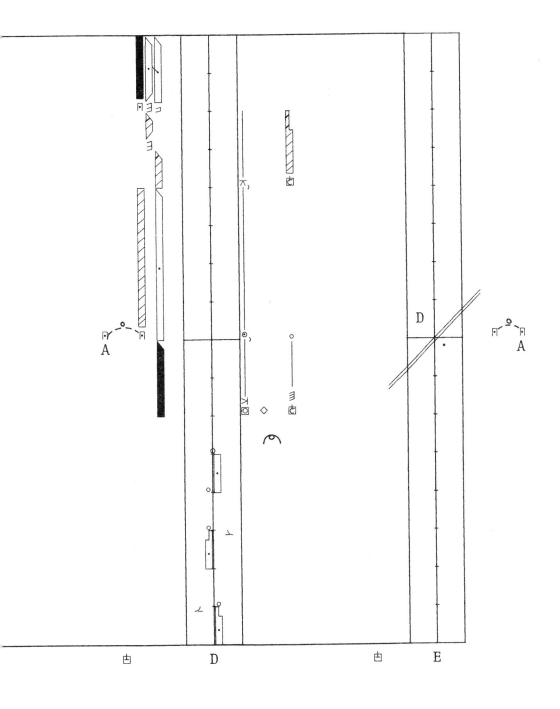

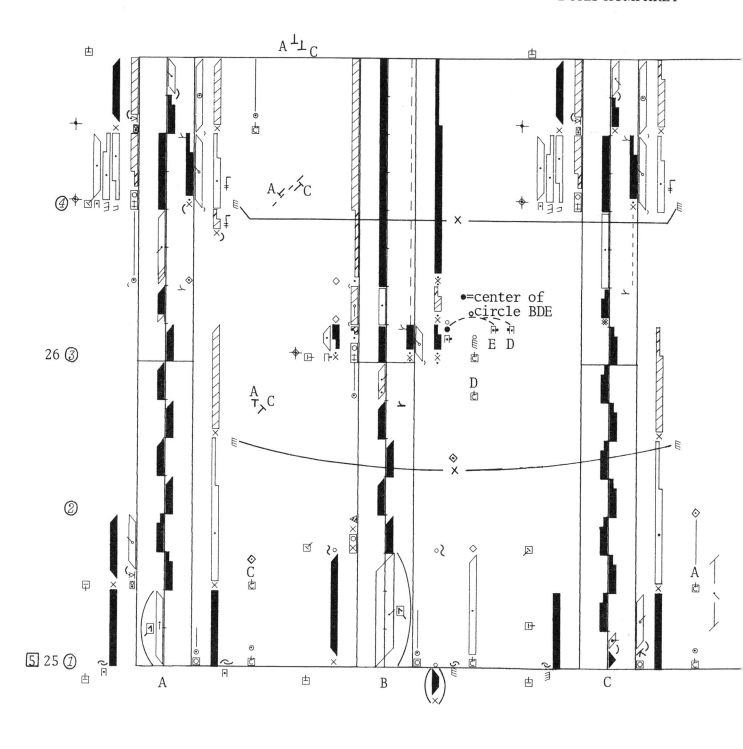

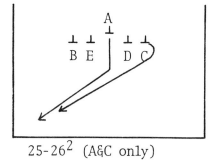

25-26² (A&C only)

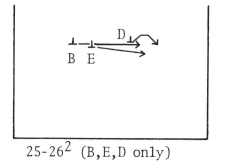

25-26² (B,E,D only)

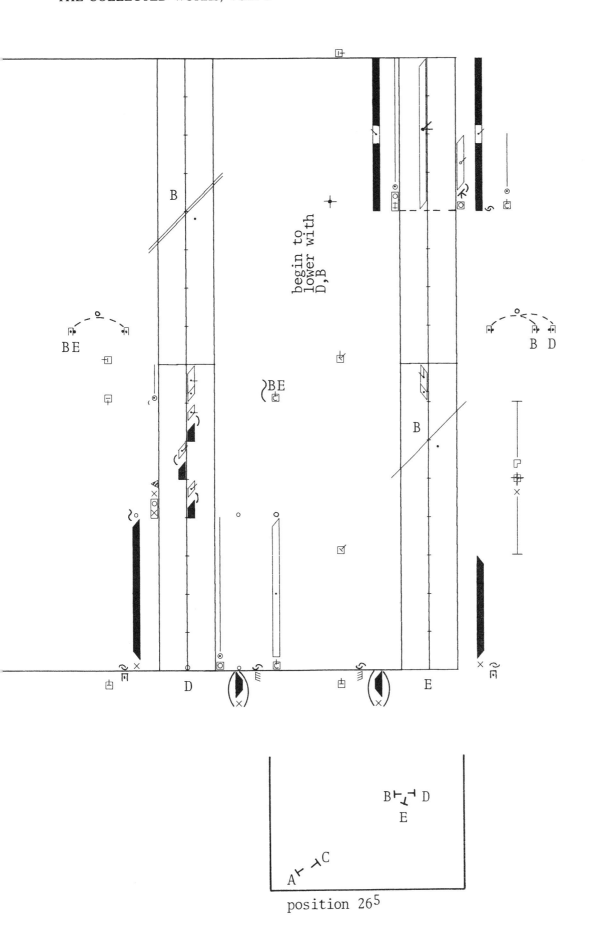

position 26⁵

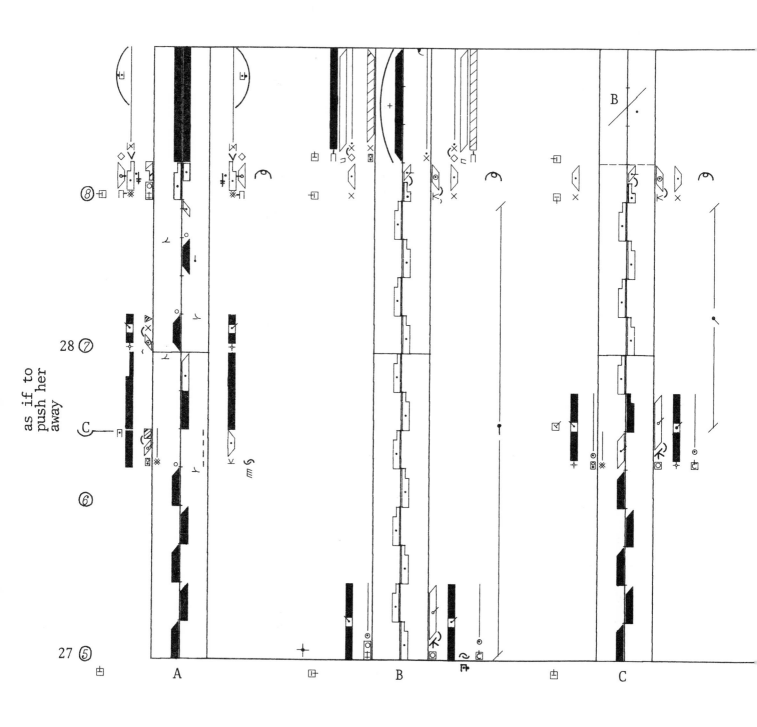

as if to
push her
away

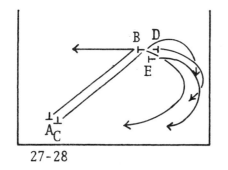

27-28

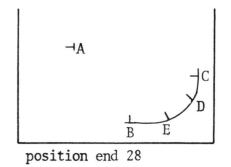

position end 28

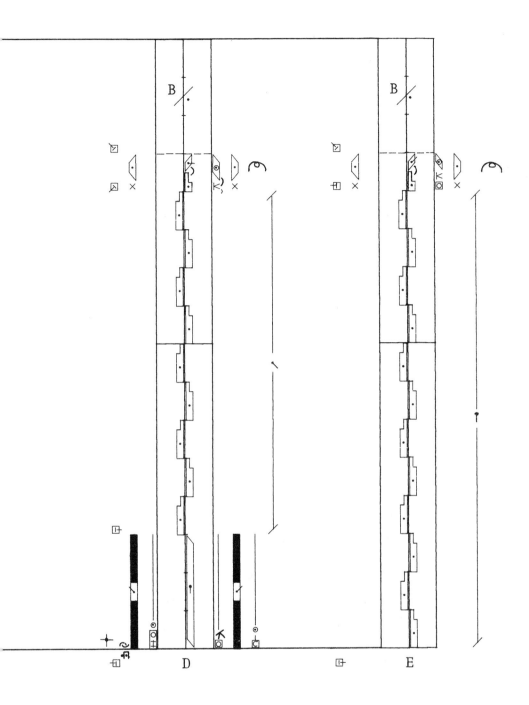

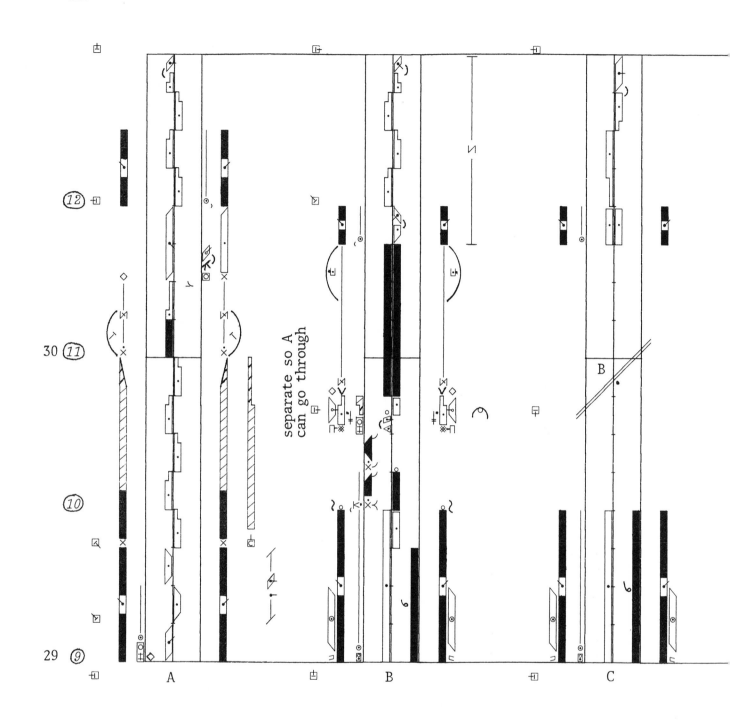

separate so A
can go through

A   B   C

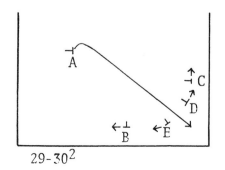

29-30²

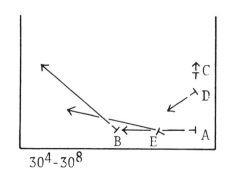

30⁴-30⁸

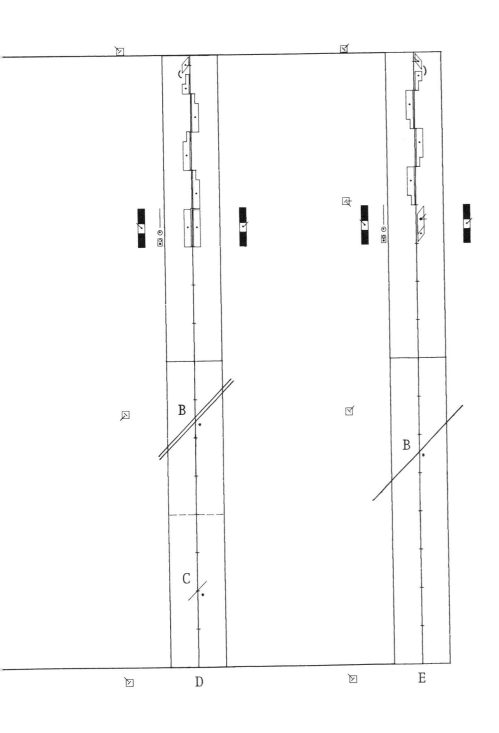

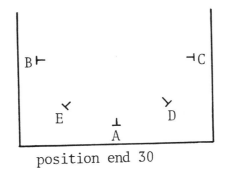

position end 30

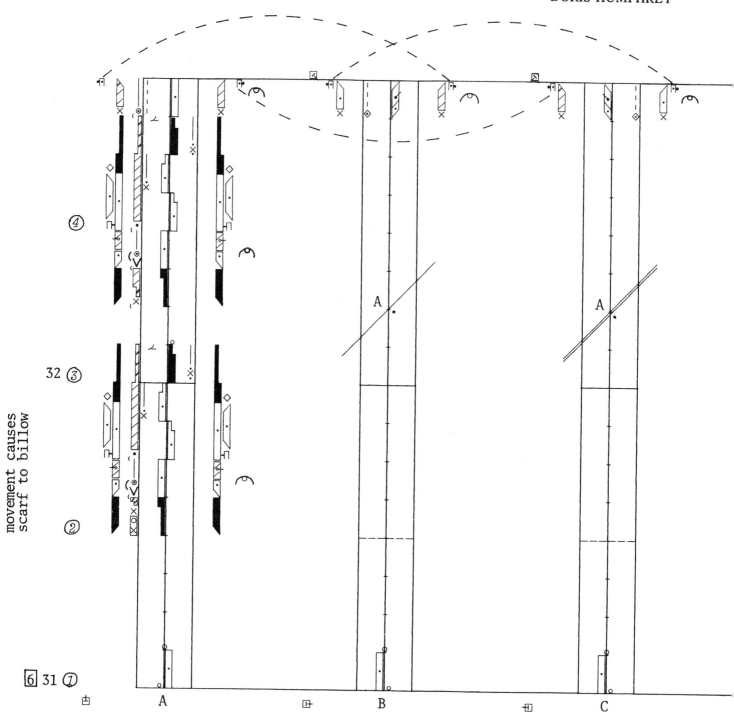

movement causes
scarf to billow

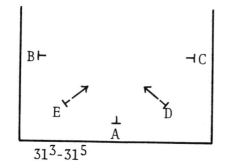

31³-31⁵

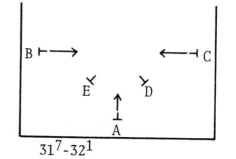

31⁷-32¹

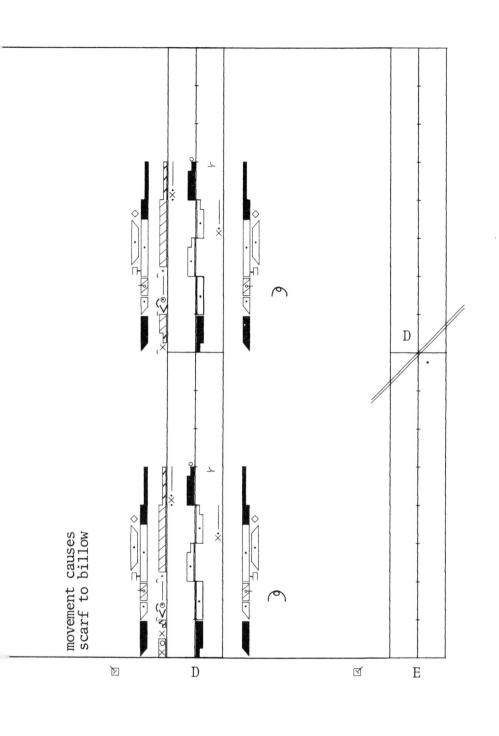

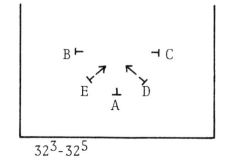

32^3-32^5

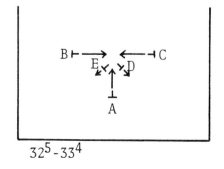

32^5-33^4

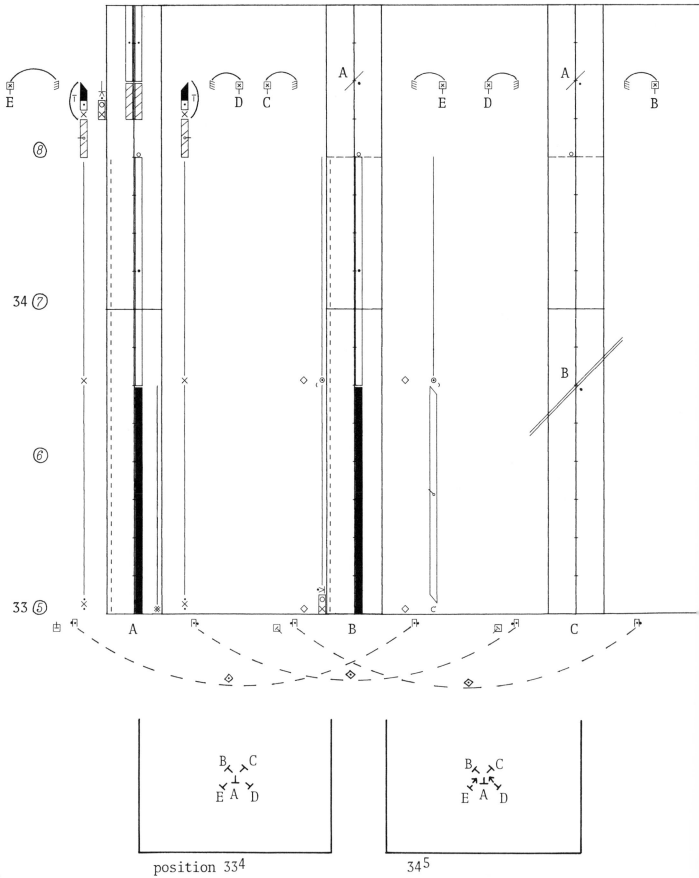

position 33⁴   34⁵

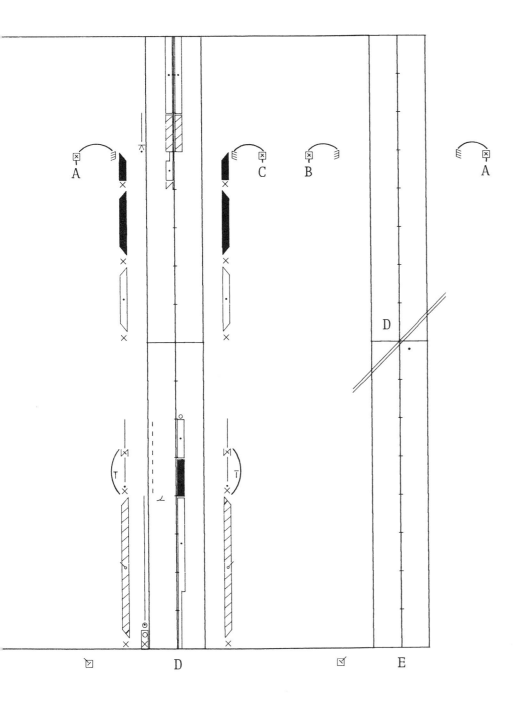

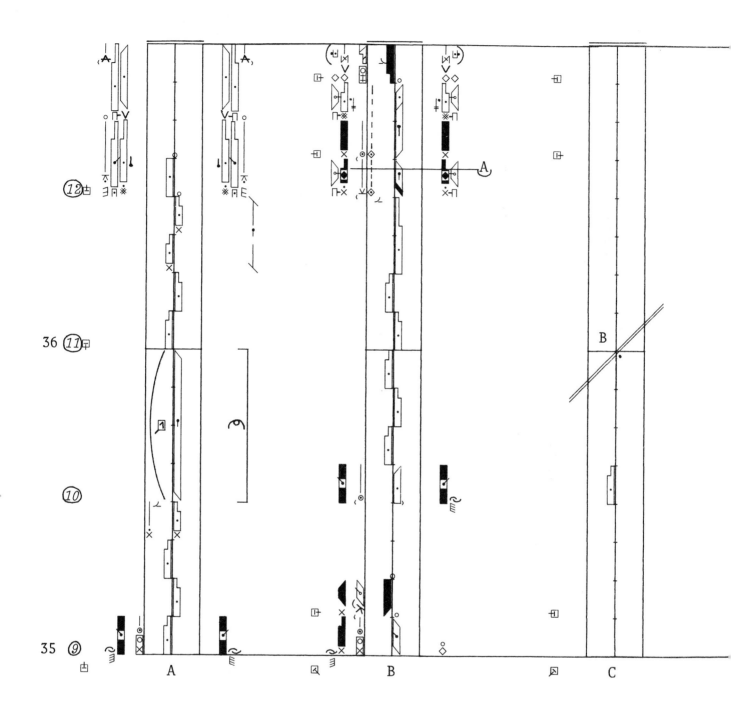

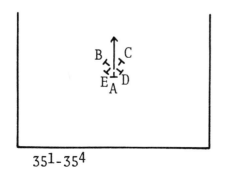

35^1–35^4

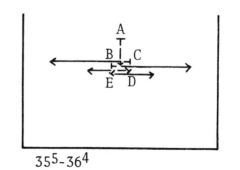

35^5–36^4

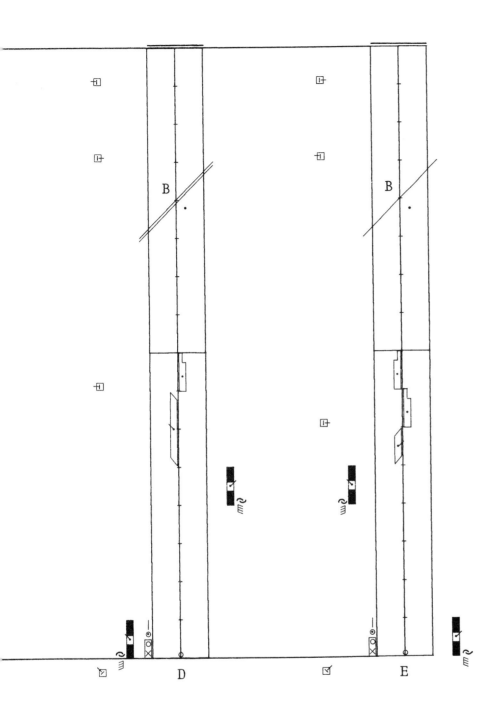

end

Two Ecstatic Themes
1. Circular Descent
2. Pointed Ascent

Choreography by
>Doris Humphrey (1931)

Taught by
>Ernestine Stodelle (1975)
>Revised (1980)

Music by
>Nicholas Medtner
>*Tragoedie-Fragment*
>>*a-moll, Op. 7, No. 2*
>G. Francesco Malipiero
>*Maschere Che Passano*

Notation by
>Jane Marriett (1975)
>Revised (1980)

Premiere: Humphrey Weidman Company, Washington Irving High School, New York, New York, October 31, 1931.

Notated Version: as taught by Ernestine Stodelle to the José Limón Dance Company, Manhattanville College, Purchase, New York, July, 1975. First performed July 19, 1975.

Running Time: "Circular Descent" - 4:32 minutes
"Pointed Ascent" - 1:48 minutes
6:20 minutes

Score checked by: Els Grelinger and Ray Cook.

Autography by: Lynne Allard.

This score was made possible, in part, by a grant from the National Endowment for the Arts, an agency of the federal government of the United States and by the generosity of the members of the Dance Notation Bureau.

This seal signifies that the notation contained in this work has been approved and meets the qualifications for a Labanotation score as set forth by the Dance Notation Bureau.

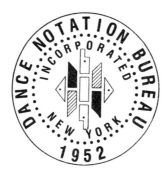

Historical Background

In a totally unexpected manner, and with the rapidity that sometimes accompanies the solution of a long-slumbering problem, Doris Humphrey clarified her creative purposes in the late spring of 1931. At the same time, a more subtle purpose was being formulated: the direction of her personal life. The solo, *Two Ecstatic Themes,* can be described as the blossoming of these two revelatory experiences.

Premiered October 31, 1931, in a joint concert with Charles Weidman at the Washington Irving High School in New York City, *Two Ecstatic Themes* was one of three new works presented on the same program. We know now that the idea for *Two Ecstatic Themes* was born independently of the music in contrast to the Bach-inspired *Air for the G String* of 1928. The story is that Doris consulted Louis Horst, her Denishawn colleague and the music director of her early concerts, with the hope of his recommending suitable music for her conception. Horst's suggestion of Nicholas Medtner's resonant *Tragoedie-Fragment* in A minor for the first theme, "Circular Descent," provided the choreographer with the perfect accompaniment for movement phrases described later in a program note as "soft and sinking, to convey an emotional feeling of acquiescence."[1] Against this quasi-abstract interpretation, Humphrey pitted her second theme, "Pointed Ascent," analyzed in the same note as moving "in pointed design to a strident climax suggestive of aggressive achievement."[2] The similarly energetic *Maschere Che Passano* I, by G. Francesco Malipiero, reflects the vigorous spirit of the contrasting "Pointed Ascent."[3]

To the dance historian, *Two Ecstatic Themes* has many tales to tell. To begin with, it represents a turning point in Doris Humphrey's career when the persistent desire to justify her use of natural movement as the basis of a dance technique was suddenly, and fully, satisfied. "I am groping for a new approach. . ." she stated in a letter to her parents in January, ten months before the premiere of the solo.[4] By mid-June, the answer lay in her hands as she read a book she had taken with her on a cruise to the Caribbean: Friedrich Nietzsche's scholarly, impassioned analysis of ancient Greek culture, *The Birth of Tragedy.*

All of Doris's previous doubts regarding the validity of her ideas concerning natural movement were swept away by Nietzsche's brilliantly conceived Apollonian-Dionysian thesis: that there exists within man himself, as exemplified by the pre-Christian Greeks, two conflicting yet intertwining impulses; namely, the desire to achieve perfection and security, and the equally compelling urge to experience the danger of the "wilder emotions."[5]

Here was the answer she had been seeking to perplexing philosophical and psychological questions that had plagued her whenever she made an attempt to analyze the most fundamental human motions: the body's resistance to gravity as expressed in the simple act of standing; the dynamics of walking and running; symmetry and asymmetry as applied to balance and imbalance; and most elusive of all, the secret wellsprings of motivation.

Translating Nietzsche's observations into movement analyses of her own, Doris Humphrey found the same quest for ecstasy in the unreality of pursuing Apollonian idealism as in ruthless Dionysian abandon. To her, the static perfection of symmetry was as congealing as the trap of total self-forgetfulness. Between these two extremes lay "the arc between two deaths,"[6] the movement realm of gravitational ebb and flow. And giving the wheel of logic one more turn, she concluded, "Fall and Recovery is the very stuff of movement."[7]

Couched in the ever-changing dynamics of Fall and Recovery, *Two Ecstatic Themes* epitomizes Doris Humphrey's credo of balance and imbalance as significant manifestations of life in action. So thorough and articulate was her kinetic transposition of Nietzsche's thesis that, at first, *Two Ecstatic Themes* was regarded in a purely academic light. John Martin's rather dry evaluation of the dance as "a study of motion applied to the simplest of ideas" (*New York Times,* November 25, 1931) was perhaps understandable, except for his disregard of the adjective "ecstatic" in the dance's title; at the time, Doris's intellectual parrying with Nietzsche was still unknown to the general public, as was also a more personal adventure that had come her way on the same Caribbean voyage. Concurrently with her discovery of the German philosopher, she had found herself — with a pleasant shock — emerging from the protective shell of her maidenhood (she was thirty-six years old at the time) as she came under the spell of a man who could arouse within her feelings of femininity never before experienced.

Charles Francis Woodford, the man whom Doris Humphrey would eventually marry, was as inspirationally responsible for the creation of *Two Ecstatic Themes* as Friedrich Nietzsche. His role, however, was to remain quietly private. Only after his wife's death and the release of their correspondence do we find proof of Doris's conversion of personal experience into dance imagery. In a letter written to her husband after a performance of the solo at

Bennington College, she declared, ". . . *our* love dance, the *Two Ecstatic Themes* made a big impression. Some of the ecstasy that was and is ours must be in it."[8]

Less direct, but equally revealing are the references found in an earlier letter written during the summer of their encounter in which Doris speaks of a "spiral curve"[9] and a "impalpable white center from which I draw new strength for work, new love for people, increased sensitivity to all things in my world."[10] Significantly, the spiral curve is the crux of the movement in "Circular Descent"; and the costume for *Two Ecstatic Themes* is pure white.

The clues were always there, but unknown at the time. Those of us who watched the premiere of Doris's new solo saw her in a new light. Here was the pristine Doris spiraling to the floor with yielding voluptuousness; and the vigor that possessed her as she fought her way upward was undeniably purposeful. Why ask for concrete references? We never sought them anyhow, knowing full well that a work of art might be inspired by self-revealing discoveries, but it is never a literal recounting of a life experience.

Only later came the program note with its philoso-phical-psychological overtones: "The whole is a counterpoint of circular and angular movement, representing the two inseparable elements of life as well as of design."[11]

Inseparable, as well, are the implications that Doris Humphrey saw fit to express in dance rather than to state in print: the curve, an ecstatic embrace, mutually protective and submissive; the angle, as assertion of self, struggling toward the ecstasy of personal fulfillment. — *E.S.*

Movement Analysis

Motivation is the all-inclusive core of dance composition, and gesture is a branch of it. [12]

Through Doris Humphrey's analysis of movement we have come to understand that motivation is subtly connected with the organic system of the human body. While the desire to move in a certain direction may be the overwhelming impulse, the gestures that a human being makes are by no means exclusively emotional or exclusively rational. Motions take place that are purely reactional: for example, the rebalancing of the body when loss of equilibrium threatens; and involuntary movements that satisfy internal needs. The entire language of Fall and Recovery is, therefore, drawn from many sources of human behavior: kinetic as well as emotional, linear as well as dynamic, irrational as well as rational.

The fact that *Two Ecstatic Themes* is a solo enables us to recognize more easily the impulse behind the various movement qualities as they occur sequentially. In the single body — the single temperament, so to speak — cadences of feeling are apt to reveal themselves more readily than in ensemble compositions which involve complex reactions. Thus, to recreate the atmosphere projected by these two exquisitely crafted dances one must study the movement as it was choreographically conceived.

The interplay between the physical act of falling/recovering and its implications as an expression of deep feeling comes to light as the curtain rises on "Circular Descent," and the dancer is discovered standing stage center, her legs planted firmly apart, her arms stretched sideways in taut, straight lines. Linearly, here is perfect symmetry; kinetically, the dancer's stance suggests absolute control; the emotional tone is one of security, of complete rationality.

With the music's first chords, the outstretched arms give way to soft curves, the breath-filled torso dips to the right and then, almost disappearing from view, it arches far backward from the thighs. A rounding out of what has become an elliptical curve now brings the dancer upward to the other side as she recovers smoothly from the imminence of a fall. The arms are now curved, one in front of the lifted body, the other to the side and slightly back. The dynamic graph of the three-dimensional movement has been clearly articulated in a purely physical sense.

But beyond the kinetic path that the dancer has traced in space, one perceives an aura of emotional enchantment. No fear of falling grips her; rather, a soft willingness to yield to the enticement of the fall seems to flow through her. Repeated three more times, the elliptical motions come to a climax with a double curve of both arms.

A strong backward pull draws her out of this suspended gesture into a turn, from which she emerges, now in profile, into a similar but higher embracing curve; and almost immediately another reverse turn swings her back with the same weighted pull that terminates with a circling of both arms overhead in a climbing spiral. As though cutting through her own enchantment, she slices downward, her right hand nearly touching the floor. The straight line has intercepted the mood — though only briefly — and the dancer returns to her original symmetrical stance.

As we shall later see, the enchantment the dancer experiences in "Circular Descent" becomes more, not less, intoxicating. It is not broken until "Pointed Ascent," when her search for equilibrium means far more than the attainment of mere stability. It is the regaining of individuality in a positive sense.

Throughout "Circular Descent," the yielding to gravity — and to love — takes the dancer on a voyage of self-discovery that, in turn, moves elliptically through space: a weaving across the stage to the high point of the "hour-glass motions"[13] and from there, into a series of backward falling steps until she has returned to the gravitational center of her first movements, now on her knees. Ecstacy is in full sway as her body draws patterned curves on the floor. A gradual return to standing, and the trance becomes complete. At the peak of a spinning turn with the arms swirling as the torso falls with astonishing abandon, the dancer suddenly stops all motion with an abrupt downward thrust of body and arm. But almost immediately she has reversed the impulse and is rising on her toes to her full height, right arm high above her head, her face and body exultantly expressive of the emotion that possesses her. Then, a slow backward fall in final ecstatic submission as the music's last chord fades into silence.

I think of dynamics as a scale extending from the smoothness of cream to the sharpness of a tack hammer.[14]

The contrasting elements between the lyrical "Circular Descent" and the dramatic "Pointed Ascent" lead us as vividly into the realm of dynamics as into the extremes of linear design.

The first series of movements has an irregular staccato accent not unlike that of a tack hammer. Abrupt shifts of weight coincide with rhythmically punctuated efforts to rise from the prone position that marked the end of "Circular Descent." A shoulder twists, an elbow is thrust upward; the head turns desperately from side to side in search of means of support; the hips pull under at a plane that gives the dancer secure positioning for subsequent attempts to rise. Gone is the luxury of sensuous suspension; everything now hangs on the thread of tenuous balance, a direct struggle against gravity and its threat of domination.

The folding and unfolding of the body in its effort to come to standing has the urgency of breath-impelled exertions. Rhythmically uneven angular thrusts end in semi-falls and near collapses. Finally, from a low crouching position that has the potential compactness of a victorious thrust, the dancer starts to pull upward with feverish, jagged accents.

In one stark second, on the last chord of the music, she strikes verticality: hands clasped high above her head, legs solidly astride.

From the foregoing descriptions, it should be apparent that the dancer who aspires to perform *Two Ecstatic Themes* should be highly skilled. The successional falls and turns in "Circular Descent" require proper placement of the pelvis at all times; and firm balance is absolutely necessary in the final spin, when the circular motion of the torso and arms is superimposed on the fast-moving body. In "Pointed Ascent," the arms must pick up the staccato accent with an alacrity comparable to fast footwork; and the thighs, taking the brunt of the levered motions, have to execute their tasks with smoothness and speed.

Above all, the would-be performer of *Two Ecstatic Themes* must be equally adept in dramatic as well as lyrical movement. "Circular Descent" and "Pointed Ascent" are theatrically rich as evocations of deep feeling. Those of us who saw Doris Humphrey perform these vibrant dances will never forget their emotional impact.

Note: I would like to express my deep gratitude to the late Charles Weidman for his approval and support of my recreation of *Two Ecstatic Themes* when I showed it to him in early July, 1975. In particular, I am most grateful for his confirmation of my interpretation of "Pointed Ascent," for which there were no notes. — *E.S.*

[1] Program, Repertory Theatre, Boston, MA, March 14-15, 1935.

[2] Ibid.

[3] The music for the recreated *Two Ecstatic Themes* was found with the assistance of the pianist-composer Vivian Fine, who was Doris Humphrey's accompanist for numerous performances of *Two Ecstatic Themes* in the 1930's.

[4] Doris Humphrey, Letter to her parents, January 16, 1931.

[5] Friedrich Nietzsche, *The Birth of Tragedy,* trans. Wm. A. Haussmann (New York: Macmillan, 1924), p. 4.

[6] Doris Humphrey, *The Art of Making Dances,* p. 106.

[7] Doris Humphrey, "My Approach to the Modern Dance," in Frederick Rand Rogers, ed., *Dance: A Basic Educational Technique* (New York: Macmillan, 1941), p. 189.

[8] Doris Humphrey, Letter to Charles Francis Woodford, no date.

[9] Doris Humphrey, Letter to Charles F. Woodford, July 21, 1931.

[10] Ibid.

[11] Program, Repertory Theatre, Boston, MA, March 14-15, 1935.

[12] Doris Humphrey, *The Art of Making Dances,* p. 112.

[13] Doris Humphrey, holograph script of "Circular Descent," reprinted in Selma Jeanne Cohen, *Doris Humphrey: An Artist First.* (Middletown, CT: Wesleyan University Press, 1972), p. 237.

[14] Doris Humphrey, *The Art of Making Dances,* p. 97.

Program Note

The following 1935 program note should be used in future programs:

Two Ecstatic Themes *is the keynote to Miss Humphrey's mature work. The first part is in circular and spiral movements, soft and sinking, to convey an emotional feeling of acquiescence. The second part, in contrast to the first, moves in pointed design to a strident climax suggestive of aggressive achievement. The whole is a counterpoint of circular and angular movement, representing the two inseparable elements of life as well as of design.*

Music

"Circular Descent" - *Tragoedie - Fragment a-moll Op. 7 No. 2*
                        by Nicholas Medtner

"Pointed Ascent" - *Maschere Che Passano*
                        by G. Francesco Malipiero

The composer Vivian Fine, who was co-pianist for performances of *Two Ecstatic Themes* with the Humphrey Weidman Company has recorded these piano pieces for the José Limón Dance Company. Copies of this recording are available from the Dance Notation Bureau.

Tempi

"Circular Descent"

Measure #	Metronome mark (♩)
1-13	begin 40, increase to 54
14	ritard
15-24	begin 40, increase to 48
25-49	begin 76, increase to 86
50	ritard (hold)
51-70	54
71-78	begin 69, increase to 160
80	ritard

"Pointed Ascent"

Measure #	Metronome mark (♩)
1-11	begin 88, increase to 97
12-16	105
17-23	96
24-25	76
26-28	96
31-36	begin 96, increase to 104
37-38	80
39-42	90

Glossary

     Movement breath - suspension with increasing lightness and sustainment -

     Falling feeling - giving in with accelerated passive weight -

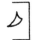   Unstretched, unbent state

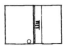   Unemphasized

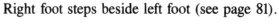   The accent applies to the entire movement.

     Direction from Body Part -
Right foot steps beside left foot (see page 81).

Left foot steps beside right foot (see page 84).

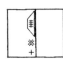   Left hip is placed slightly to the side of where feet were (see page 86).

The torso movements in "Circular Descent" have been written with ▯ because the Humphrey technique involves a strong pelvic-thigh connection. When this connection is used, the performance of these circular torso paths does not strain the lower back, but works the thigh-pelvis connection.

Standard retention (see Knust's *A Dictionary of Kinetography Laban*, D 217i)

The relationship of the body part to the standard system of reference (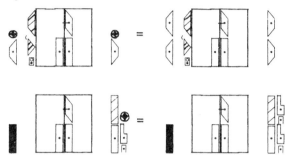) does not change. In other words, repeat the previous direction symbol.

See page 73, m. 20 - arms remain side middle from

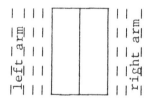

Arm columns for "Circular Descent"

measure #   1

section #   ☐

dancer's counts   ①

2)

3)

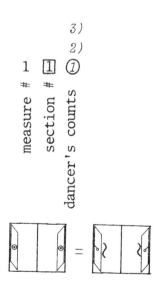

"Circular Descent"

Measures 1-8	Timing of phrases (6 counts) is not exact timing, phrases should swing. Feel the edge of the kinesphere with your head. Arms are shaping (carving) because the body makes them. The arms envelop the space. The head should disappear at the back of the swoon. There should be a feeling of suspension from the chest and a lift in the upper back at the back of the swoon. The front of the hips should feel elongated. To assist the swoon, allow the knee to go forward.
Measures 5-8	Deeper, broader than the first phrase, feel a bit beyond the kinesphere.
Measure 8	Imagine that you see a lover, whom you embrace. Scoop the arms together.
End of Measure 10	Keep the shape and pull with the right hip to make the turn in measure 11.

 A black space hold placed within a direction symbol indicates moving with undeviating aim to the direction indicated. The direction is judged from the end of the accompanying turn. (See page 73, m. 23.)

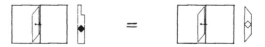

Track Pins

Track pins are used to indicate relationship to the center lines of the body. Track pins used next to a direction symbol indicate how the direction is to be modified into five tracks.

The five tracks in the sagittal direction are:

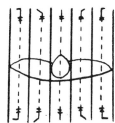

solid lines = division of tracks

dotted lines = center line of each track

When these pins are used to modify a direction symbol, the extremity is on the center line of that particular track.　⊥　is the normal, un-written track for the left arm when moving sagittally,　⌊　for the right arm.　⊥　expresses the exact center line of the body. The use of a dot to modify the track pin indicates that the extremity is in the track but not on the center line; it is slightly to one side.

⋅⊥　= slightly to the left of the center line of the body

⊥⋅　= slightly to the right of the center line of the body

For example:

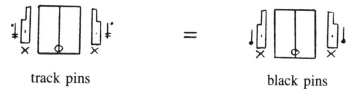

track pins　　　　　　　　　　　　　　black pins

As of 1981, the use of track pins has been explored only for the arms. They may not as yet be used for the legs. For further information, including a discussion of diagonal and lateral tracks, see either *Teachers' Bulletin,* Number 6, May, 1980, (copies available at the Dance Notation Bureau, New York) or the 1979 I.C.K.L. papers.

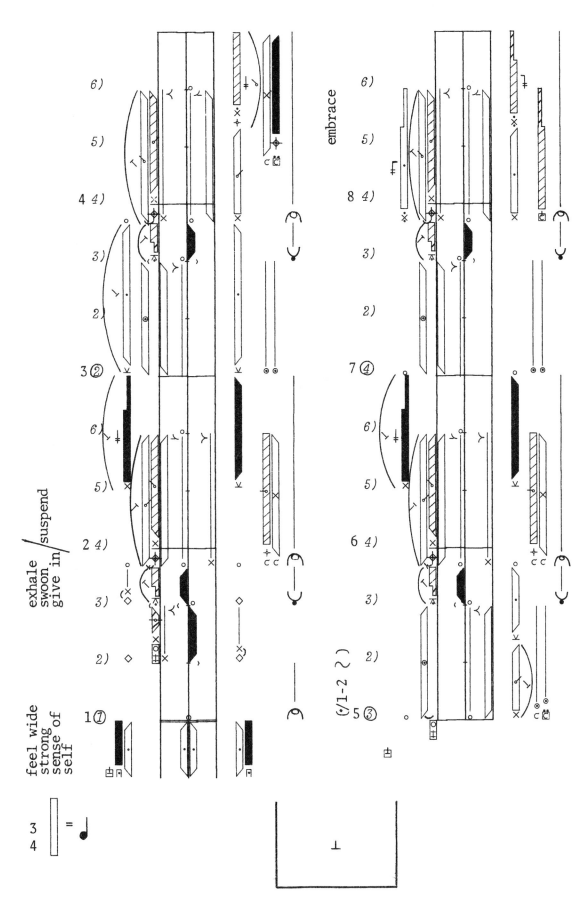

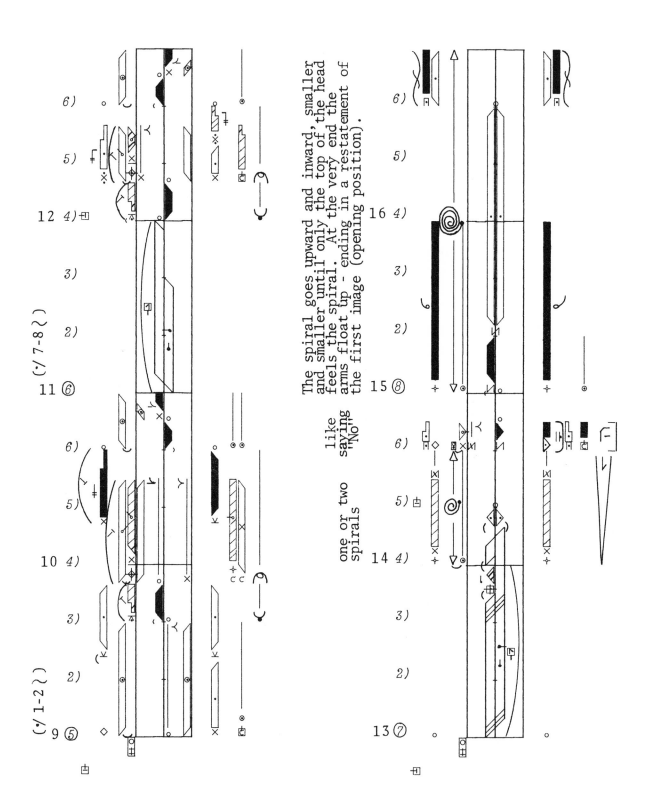

The spiral goes upward and inward, smaller and smaller until only the top of the head feels the spiral. At the very end the arms float up - ending in a restatement of the first image (opening position).

like saying "No"

one or two spirals

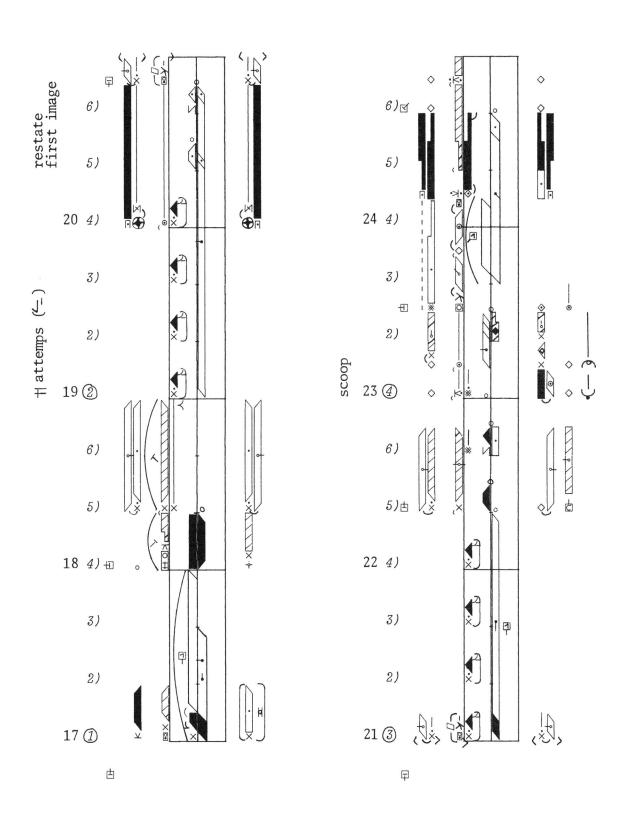

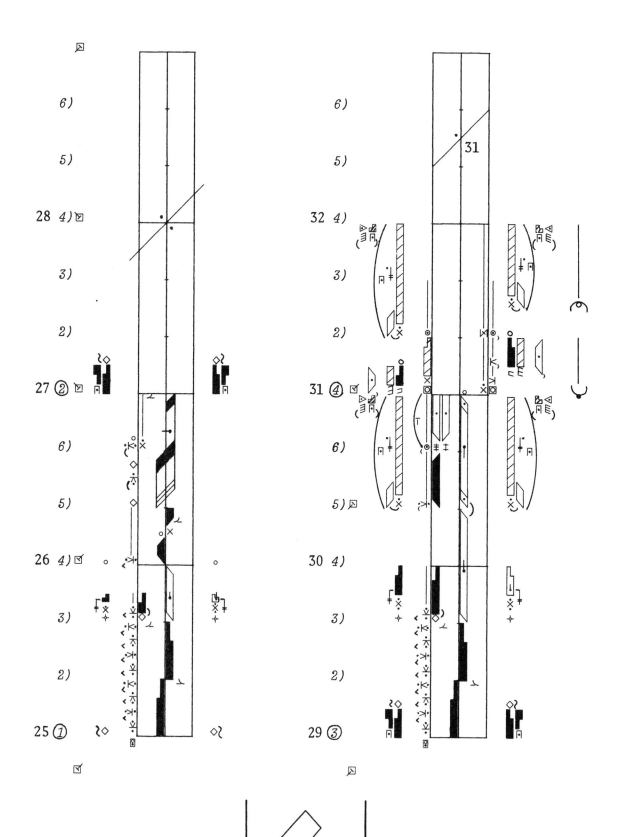

25-29

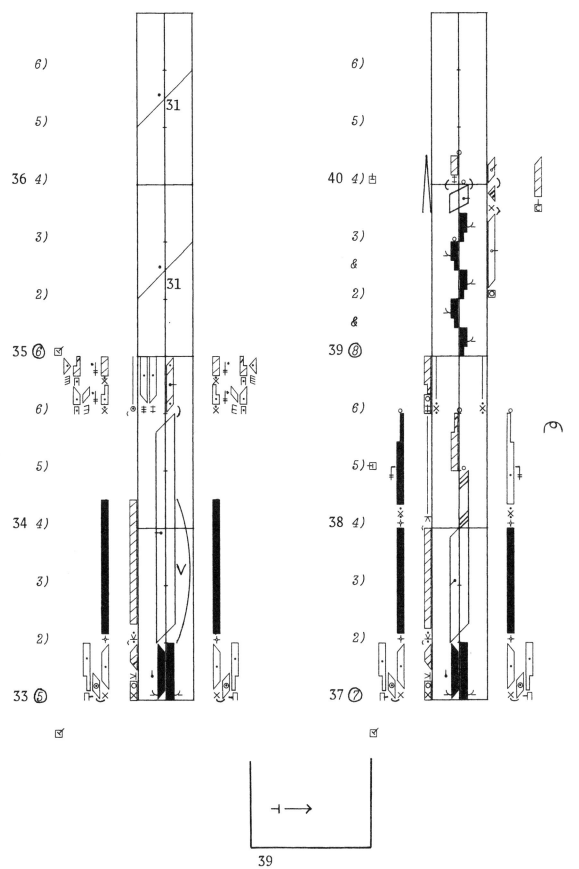

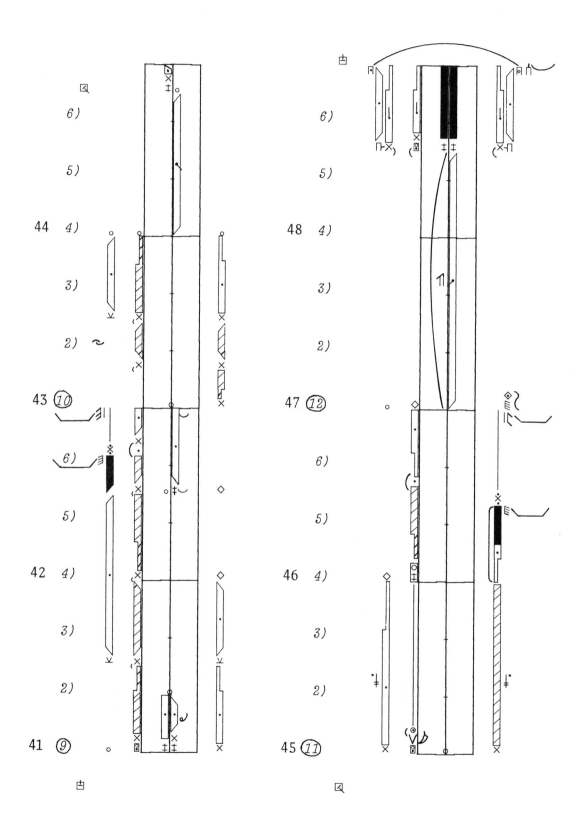

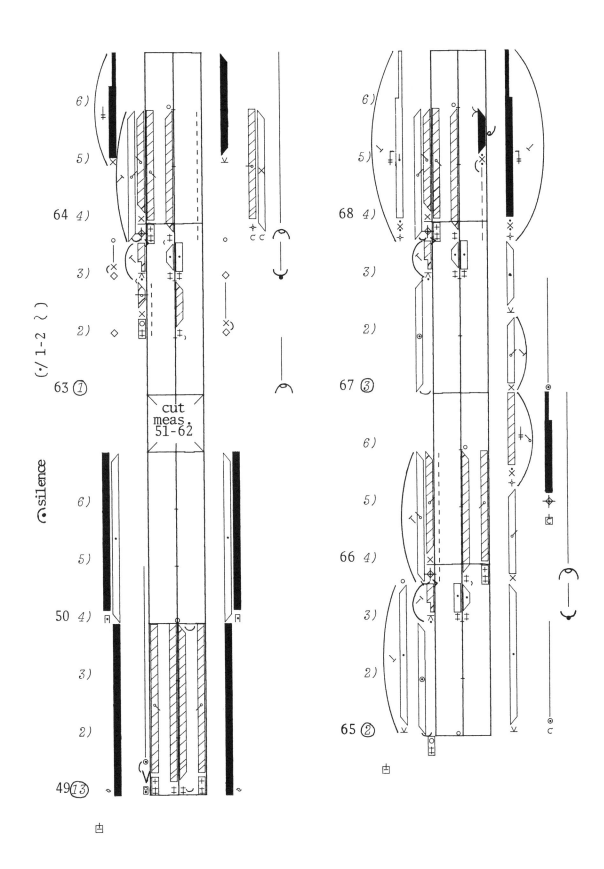

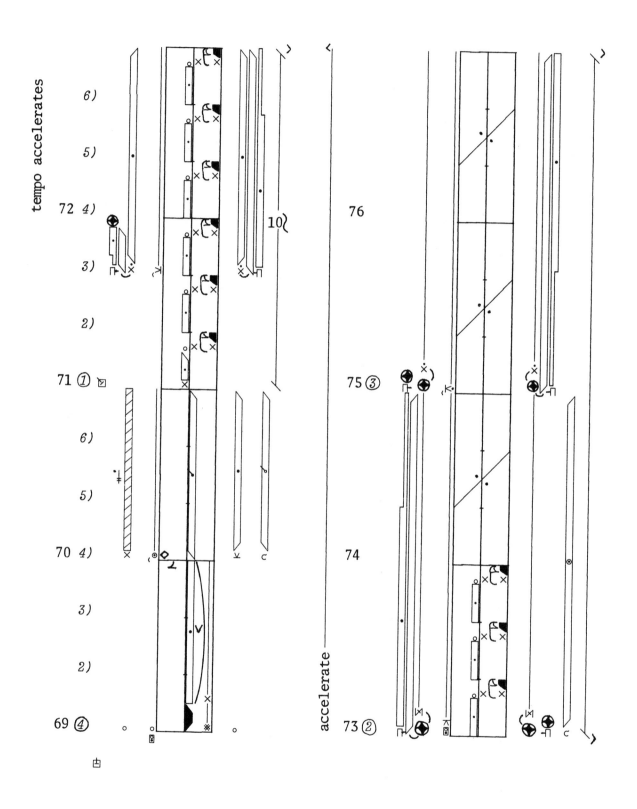

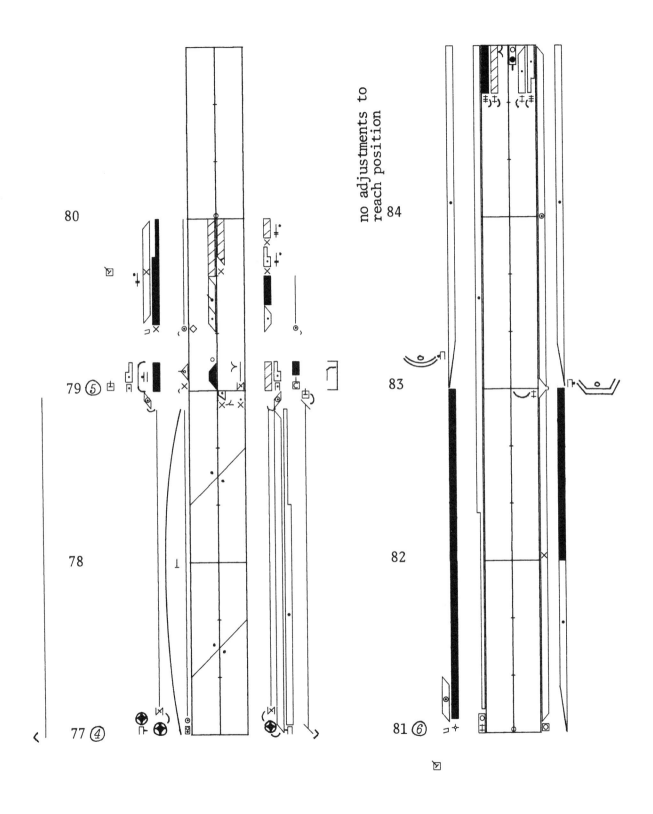

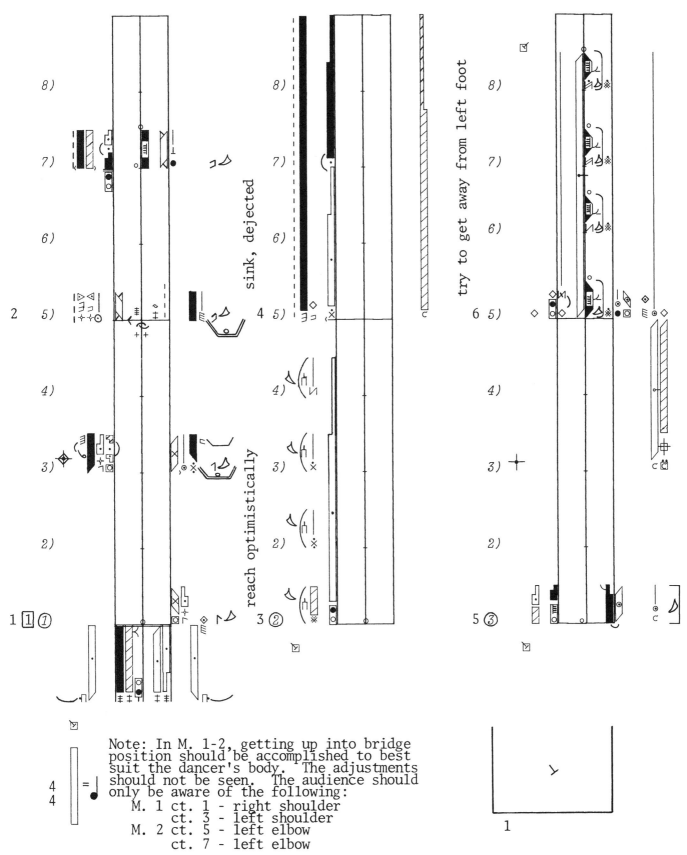

sink, dejected

reach optimistically

try to get away from left foot

Note: In M. 1-2, getting up into bridge
position should be accomplished to best
suit the dancer's body. The adjustments
should not be seen. The audience should
only be aware of the following:
    M. 1 ct. 1 - right shoulder
         ct. 3 - left shoulder
    M. 2 ct. 5 - left elbow
         ct. 7 - left elbow

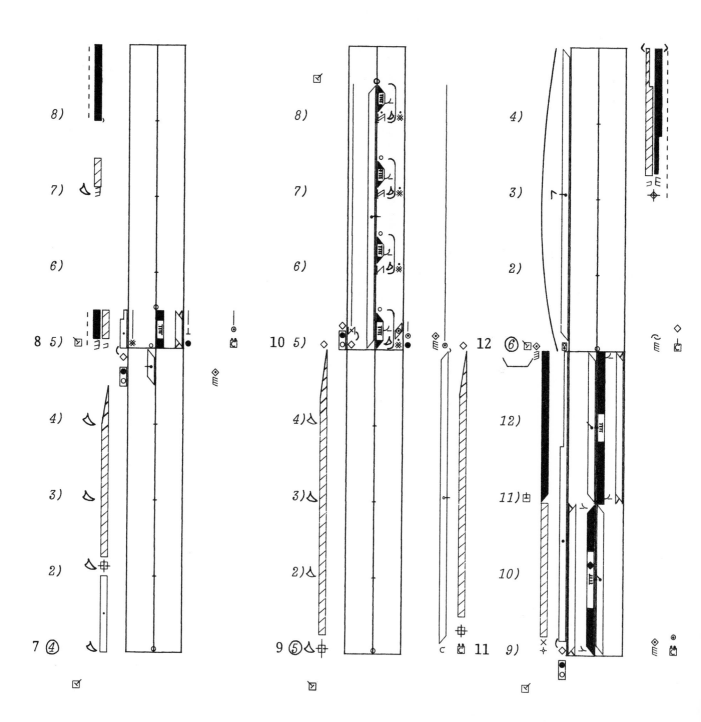

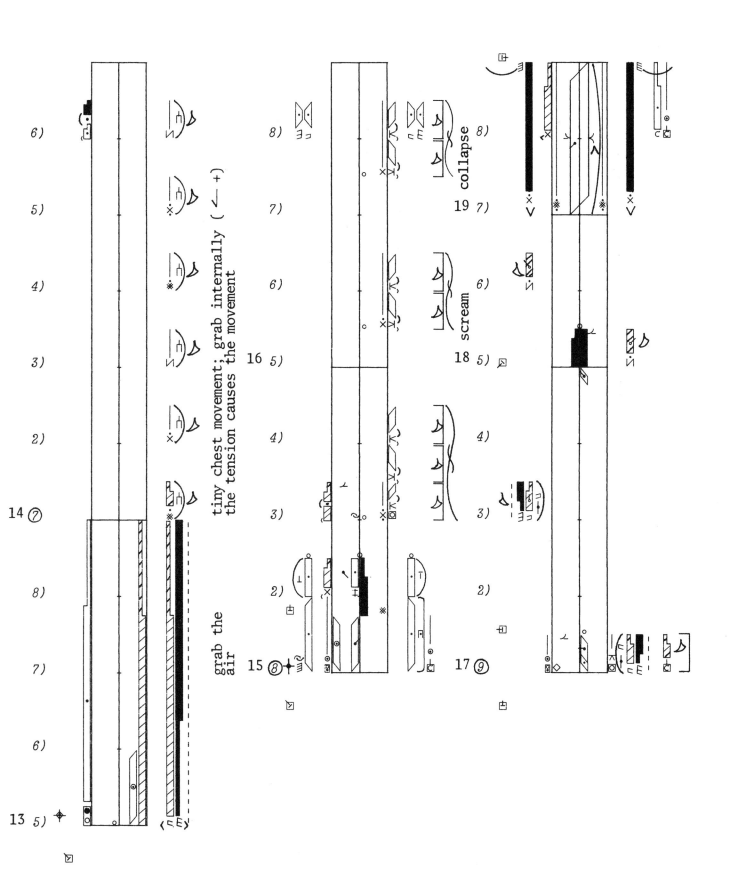

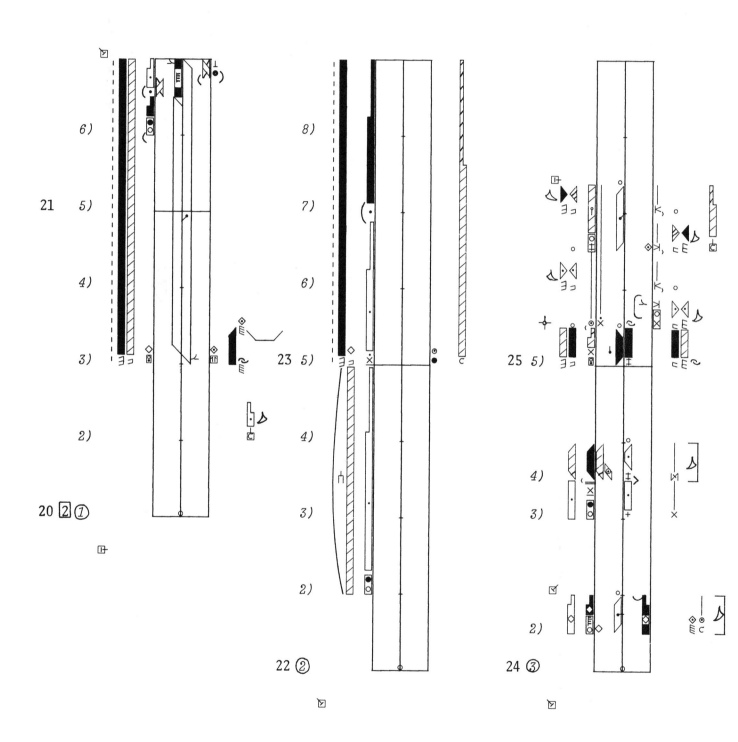

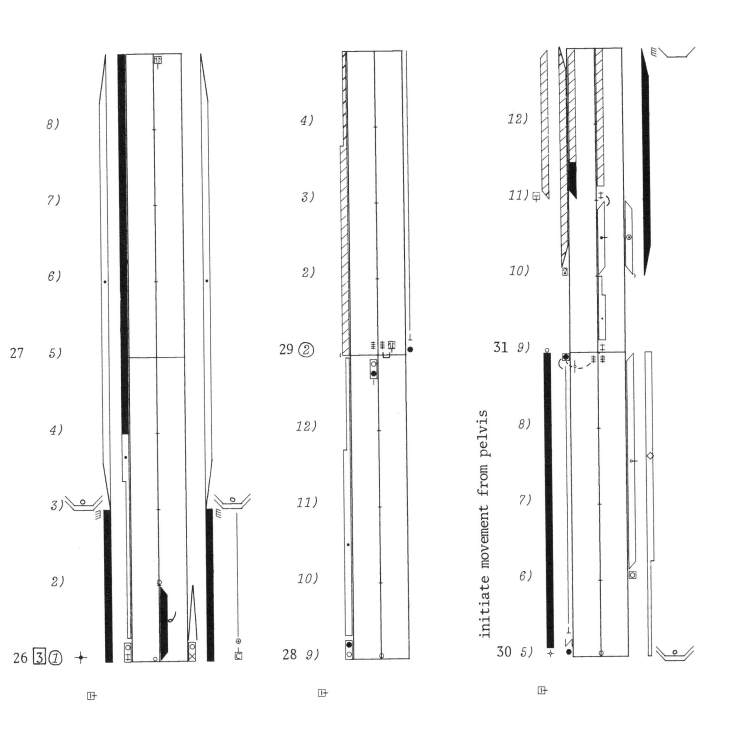

initiate movement from pelvis

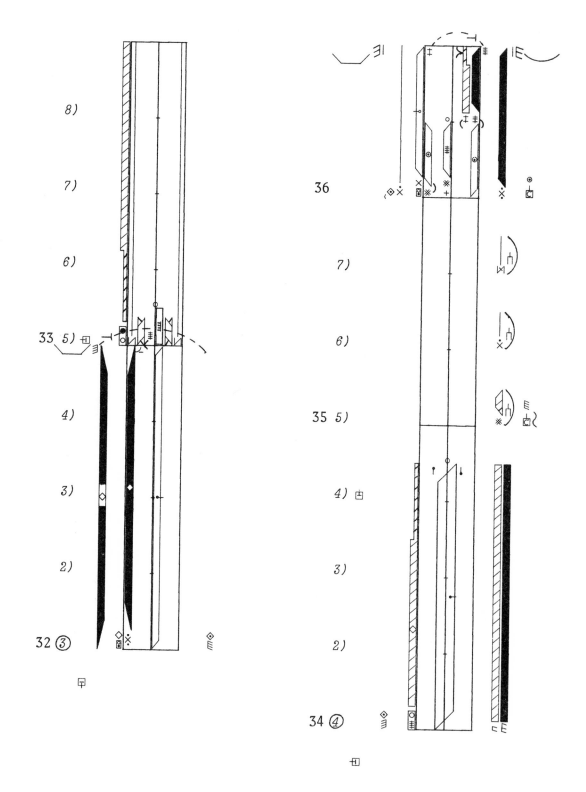

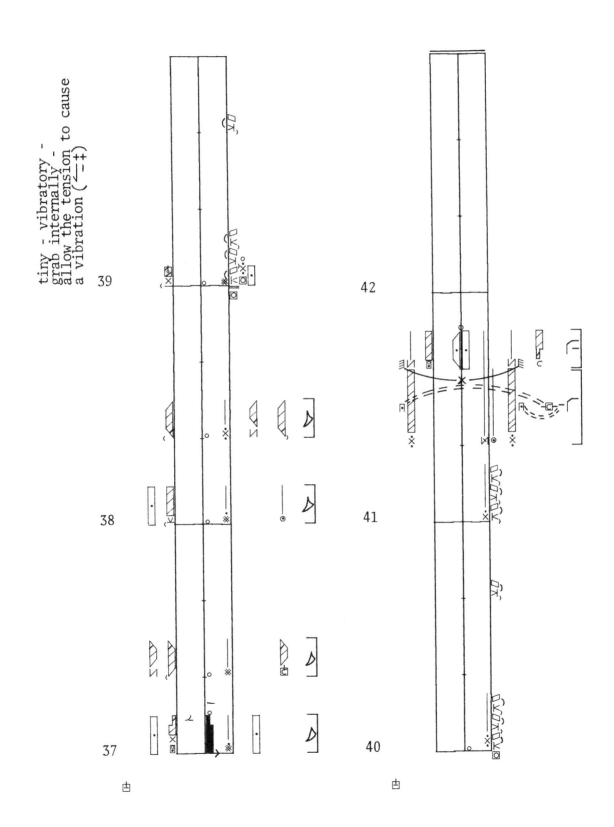

Day on Earth

Choreography by
Doris Humphrey (1947)

Music by
Aaron Copland (1941)
Piano Sonata

Notation by
Muriel Topaz (1959)
Revised (1978 & 1981)

Boston Premiere: May 10, 1947 at Beaver Country Day School by the Jose Limon Dance Company.

NY Premiere: December 21, 1947, at the New York City Center by the Jose Limon Dance Company.

Notated Version: As performed by the Jose Limon Dance Company at Connecticut College, August, 1959.

Running Time: Approximately 20 minutes.

Score Checked by: Jane Marriett.

Autography by: Lynne Allard.
Additional Autography by: Letitia Coburn.

This score was made possible by funds from the Doris Humphrey Memorial Fund, and is the property of the Fund, which is administered by the Lincoln Center Library for the Performing Arts.

The notation was updated and minor revisions made in 1978 with funds from the National Endowment for the Arts, a federal agency, and from funds raised by the Dance Notation Bureau at the 50th Anniversary Doris Humphrey Celebration. The revisions were made by the original notator. Further revisions were made in 1981 based on comments by Lucy Venable who worked with the score and the original silent film (made at Connecticut College by Helen Priest Rogers). Ms. Venable's comments were made in conjunction with her restaging of the work at The Ohio State University, 1979-1980. Subsequently, minor corrections were added after various stagings by Ms. Venable and Letitia Coburn.

The notator wishes to thank Ms. Venable, Ms. Coburn, Ruth Currier and Letitia Ide for their invaluable comments on the score.

This seal signifies that the notation contained in this work has been approved and meets the qualifications for a Labanotation score as set forth by the Dance Notation Bureau.

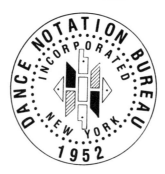

90

Historical Background

In a letter written less than nine months after the premiere of *Day on Earth*, Doris Humphrey describes her newest work: ". . . it's about the family, and employs a little girl of eleven." Then she adds, "Almost all modern dance has gone psychopathic so this is a really daring piece because, although a tragedy, it is healthy!"[1]

It was indeed daring in 1947 to create a dramatic ballet that dealt only with natural, easily recognizable events in a man's life. Such simplicity of expression was not in vogue at a time when plots had to be thickened with what Doris Humphrey called "a touch of arsenic"[2] to be palatable. But how true to Doris's personality was the need to invest narrative with philosophy rather than to interpret human action solely from a psychological point of view. Time and again we have seen her lift a storyline out of literal sequence into universal terms. The early *Shakers* (1930), with its religious fervor, and the Cretan-inspired *Dionysiagues* (1932), with its pagan ritual, bear testimony to the choreographer's ability to project a theme beyond the specifics of history, geography, or personal psychology. Likewise, the affirmative visions of the later *New Dance* (1936) and *Passacaglia* (1938) stood for "the world as it should be, where each person has a clear and harmonious relationship to his fellow beings."[3] Here was philosophy at its loftiest, and, we might add, dance at its purest.

This is not to say that Doris Humphrey was indifferent to the power of the subconscious. Her written statements, "A movement without a motivation is unthinkable"[4] and "It is probably rare for a choreographer deliberately to make a choice of a theme by rational means"[5] prove, as well as did her dramatically stirring *With*

My Red Fires (1936), that Doris Humphrey was acutely aware of the irrational side of man's nature and knew how to deal with it on the stage. Basically, however, Doris was an extrovert, a realistically minded person who could come to grips with the immediacies of life and still arrive at the larger view.

That Doris Humphrey was a realist in theatrical matters became apparent in the summer of 1946 when she was asked by José Limón to become Artistic Director of a small, newly organized ensemble, actually the outgrowth of a trio he had formed the preceding spring with Dorothy Bird and Beatrice Seckler. Hitherto, the strongest impulse in Doris's creative life had been to compose for large groups of dancers. Such preferences had been reluctantly abandoned in 1945 when the misfortunes of a more and more incapacitating arthritis coincided with the unfeasibility of maintaining the sizeable Humphrey-Weidman Company. (Nor would those preferences surface again until Martha Hill would perceptively invite her nearly a decade later to establish the Juilliard Dance Theatre).

For a choreographer of less resourcefulness, working with a mere handful of dancers after the gratifications of directing a large ensemble might have ended in fruitless compromise. But the realistic bent of Doris's mind adjusted itself with positive enthusiasm. And why not? With his war years behind him, the promising José was laying his future in her hands; and alongside of him were two women of longtime association in whom she had utmost confidence: the versatile Beatrice Seckler and the statuesque, expressive Letitia Ide.

Her first compositions, a farcical duo for Limón and Seckler, *The Story of Mankind,* and the elegiac *Lament for Ignacio Sanchez Meijas* with Limón, Ide, and the actress, Ellen Love, successfully launched the company at Bennington College in Vermont.

Within months, a talented young girl named Miriam Pandor and a winsome child, Melissa Nicolaides, would be conjoined with Limón and Ide to form the cast of *Day on Earth*. And in less than two years, José's small group would be reinforced by the virtuosic Pauline Koner and a progression of superbly gifted performers — Betty Jones, Ruth Currier and Lucas Hoving — who would constitute, by 1949, a chamber ensemble *extraordinaire*. But not before *Day on Earth* had made its mark in the annals of modern dance as one of Doris Humphrey's finest compositions, did critic John Martin exclaim, ". . . we have not begun to realize her true stature."[6]

Set to Aaron Copland's stringently structured *Piano Sonata, Day on Earth* is a masterfully conceived tribute to the family as an ongoing unit of natural life. The action spans a man's existence, presumably a farmer's, from youth through maturity. Its three sections are choreographically entitled "Man's Work and First Love," "The Family" and "Loss, and the Refuge of Work."

The wholesome experiences of tilling the soil, reaping its goodness, and of finding (and losing) young love comprise the man's early experiences. When mature love enters, a new era begins: marriage and with it the joys of parenthood. This, too, ends in loss, for the child inevitably leaves. Distraught, the mother cannot be comforted; her grief culminates in death; in tortured despair the man seeks solace in his work. The final moments convey the radiance of resignation as the man moves quietly into the folds of death himself, surrounded by memories of his wife, his first sweetheart, and his child who physically reenter in the form of visions. The voluminous silk scarf that had symbolically covered the child at birth is now drawn over the recumbent forms of the man and his two loves. Seated above them, the child gazes confidently into the future of her own day on earth.

Typical of Doris Humphrey's compositional subtleties, the characters in *Day on Earth* were delicately etched, not literally drawn. Typical, also, was her choreographic sharing, in which she encouraged participatory inventiveness on the part of her cast. Letitia Ide as the Wife-Mother created whole passages of movement in response to Doris's evocative directives. Ruth Currier, who replaced Miriam Pandor, translated the choreographer's rhythmic suggestions into eloquent sequences of her own that gave her, without explicit analyses on Humphrey's part, the "inner motivations"[7] of the "untamed"[8] girl she portrayed. Watching in fascination as Doris rehearsed the child, whom she wanted to behave spontaneously rather than perform like a trained dancer, Currier remembers hearing Doris call out suggestively, "Pick cherries . . . follow the snake . . . play hide and seek . . . skip over there!"[9] And both dancers recall Doris's long sessions with Jose. "She was tough on him. He could take it."[10] Their dual struggle to achieve perfection would be relentless.

Inspired by, but rising above the individualities of its performers, *Day on Earth* discloses none of the meanness of man, only the grand scheme of simple lives lived in accordance with nature's everlasting cycle of birth and death. — *E.S.*

Movement Analysis

The emotional rhythm may be cast into a breath rhythm, a motor rhythm or gestural sequences. [11]

When the curtain rises on *Day on Earth*, a patch of light falls on the figure of a man in the right upstage corner. He is about to advance with plowing and seeding motions along a narrow path that leads diagonally downstage. Another patch of light picks up a female group barely left of upstage center. A square-shouldered woman is seated on a box, legs quite widely placed, arms resting on the thighs with one hand turned up, the other down. At the woman's feet is a soft mound made by the folds of a large silk scarf (it covers the form of a child). Standing next to her is a slender girl, youthful in manner and build. "The female group should have, Doris told us, the quality of a Henry Moore family statue."[12]

With the first slow bars of the music, the man proceeds downstage with his earth-related motions, unaware of the presence of the two women until the young girl impetuously runs across the stage and drops softly into a fall. Responding to her beauty and charm, he dances with her at first lightly and joyously, and then with increasing desire. During their dance, the woman continues to look out as though gazing into the far future. When the girl, not yet ready to commit herself, leaves the scene, and the man returns to his tasks, the woman rises and slowly spreads open the scarf that had partially covered the child.

This whole part should have the joy of the beginning of a great love, plus the euphoria of a most perfect summer day. The two sharp accents with the right arm should have an ecstatic quality, which is also in the two turns moving forward with arms overhead, alive with in-out breath pulse. A rich, warm, rounded style is called for throughout. At the end of their duet, the man and the woman join hands in a kind of marriage pledge, turn and move upstage in the silence between the first and second movements of the music and approach and awaken the child.

What is this "rich, warm, rounded style" but the movement quality of those whose sense of faith in each other and in their environment is rich, warm, and rounded? The woman's family is her citadel; her trust in the love she receives is unquestioning. Her gestures are directly expressive of her uncomplicated emotions.

The second movement, sometimes called *The Family*, has periods of play interspersed with work movements of the parents. There is even a moment when the mother slips away, and the child feels temporarily lost; but she turns to the father and establishes a happy relationship with him before the mother's return. A note of foreboding is introduced when, after the final game the threesome play.

The child drops out of the little up-and-down jumps sooner than the others, and the mother makes two encircling arm movements toward the child, both unsuccessful, thus turning the game into sad reality. The child then rises from a final crouching position with ever so slow alternating arm circles denoting the passage of time, and moves offstage, eyes on the parents, left hand lifted in farewell. Moving slowly, steadily downstage on the opposite side, the parents sink to the floor.

Here is more than a simple farewell. A whole life seems to be at stake; and though the reason for the child's leavetaking is not clear, the parents' suffering is acute. With the beginning of the third movement, the woman's sorrow mounts uncontrollably.

Her lament is a combination of movements of anguish with sharp arm thrusts in turns or slanted in the direction of the child's departure; also, slow, sorrowful stretching movements with twisted breath releases, like cries coming from the solar plexus. There are searching, confused, and desperate moments when the mother almost hysterically seeks to find the child again.

The man is supportive of the woman for most of the lament, but at the end, when she breaks away from him and runs upstage in desperation, I felt a sense of conflict.

The man's tightly wound movements, beating feet, wildly striking arms and abrupt jumps have a frenzied thrust. Then calm returns as he resolutely resumes his plowing, seeding movements. In a moment of suspended wonder, he watches the woman lift the scarf from the box and begin the slow, sustained ritual of its folding, an act that suggests that she is preparing for her own death.

"This whole sequence [with the scarf] should be almost continuous, smoothly moving with only two small accents: folding the scarf down over the chest, and finally folding it high in the air before lowering oneself to the box as life seems to drain out to the earth."

Ide concludes: "The very last section should have a dream-like, other-worldly, floating quality, as though propelled by spirit (not muscle)."

With the last bars of the music, the man, the woman and the young girl settle back underneath the outspread scarf as the child, seated squarely on the box, faces the dawning of her own day on earth. — *E.S.*

[1] Doris Humphrey, Letter to author, February 1, 1948.

[2] Doris Humphrey, Letter to Helen Mary Robinson, no date. Quoted in Selma Jeanne Cohen, *Doris Humphrey: An Artist First*, p. 192.

[3] Doris Humphrey papers, no date. Doris Humphrey Collection, Dance Collection, New York Public Library for the Performing Arts.

[4] Doris Humphrey, *The Art of Making Dances*, p. 110.

[5] Ibid., p. 32.

[6] *New York Times*, 4 January 1948.

[7] Interview with Ruth Currier, May 10, 1983.

[8] Ibid.

[9] Ibid.

[10] Interviews with Ruth Currier, Letitia Ide, May, July, 1983.

[11] Doris Humphrey, *The Art of Making Dances*, p. 108.

[12] This quotation and those that follow are taken from a description of the action in *Day on Earth* by Letitia Ide, who danced in the premiere. The author wishes to express her indebtedness to Miss Ide and to Muriel Topaz, notator of the score of *Day on Earth*, for the insights afforded in the study of the role of the Woman on which this movement analysis is mainly based.

Original Cast

Man (Farmer)   -   José Limón
Young Girl   -   Miriam Pandor
Woman   -   Letitia Ide
Child   -   Melissa Nicolaides

Notated Version Cast

J - Man (Farmer) - José Limón
R - Young Girl   - Ruth Currier
L - Woman   - Letitia Ide
C - Child   - Abigail English

Casting Information

J — A strong very masculine figure; a farmer. The role requires a
     virtuoso performer with technical security, great stamina, and
     a strong, dramatic persona.

L — A large, earthy, mature dancer, an earth mother figure with great
     dramatic projection.

R — An "air" dancer, light, young, quick, a jumper. R is a bit
     troubled, as are most adolescents, but she must take the stage
     like a spring shower.

C — A pre-pubescent child 8-10 years old, but as young looking as
     possible. A good imagination and fine musicality are more
     necessary than technical skills.

Notes on the Notation

This dance was notated after Miss Humphrey's death, performed by dancers who, with the exception of the child, have performed the work for many years and who have made the roles very much their own; therefore, the score tends to be reflective of their performances, and should be reconstructed with this in mind.

Film Information

A film of the dance is housed at the Dance Notation Bureau. The film, which has also been transferred to VHS videotape, is silent, black and white 16mm and was made at Connecticut College in 1959. The cast is the same as that of the notated version of this dance. The versions are quite similar but not identical.

There is also a version of the above film at the Dance Collection, New York Public Library for the Performing Arts (NYPL) containing music dubbed in later. The dubbing was done under the supervision of José Limón and Ruth Currier. The music was recorded and dubbed several years after the film was made, thus adjustments were made mechanically to make the two fit. The coordination of music and dance are as accurate as can be expected under the circumstances, but cannot be relied upon as a guide to detailed coordination of the two.

Another film, 16mm color, made at The Juilliard School from a production directed by José Limón is housed at the Dance Collection, NYPL.

Music Information

The music score is available through Boosey & Hawkes, 24 E. 21st Street, New York, NY.

There is no commercial recording suitable for the dance.

Props

BOX

= Box

The box is painted battleship grey. The approximate proportions of the box are:

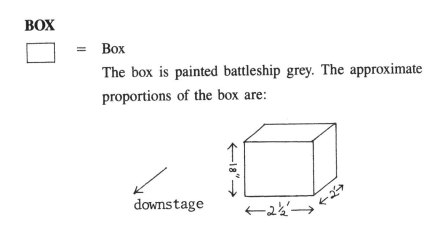

Placement of the box: The box is placed upstage and slightly left of center so that near the end of the dance, when L gets up and walks forward, (Bar 157), she is center stage.

CLOTH

= Cloth (or scarf)

The cloth is made of China silk in approximately these proportions:

(Note: China silk not crepe de chine)

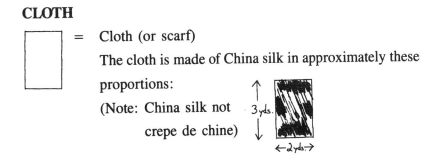

The length is measured by doubling the length from L's nose to the floor. The width is measured from L's fingertip to fingertip when she has her arms outstretched in second position.

The cloth is dyed in blended colors, going from soft yellow to orange to brown. It is also splattered with paint, but very lightly. The darkest places are the ends and, to help L find the middle, there are dark splotches at the middle of each side. Bastings and/or safety pins are also placed at the middle to help L find middle for folding. Each corner should be a slightly different color from the others.

As the dance opens, the cloth is covering the child who is lying on the floor in front of the box. Note that the child's head is not covered. L, who is seated on the box, is holding the two upstage ends of the cloth. The cloth is resting on L's knees; the left corner folded up on top of the cloth, the right corner folded under the cloth, i.e.,

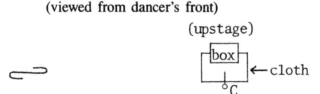

L lays the cloth on the bench shortly after she begins to dance.

At the beginning of the second movement, L picks up the downstage edge of the cloth and folds it back to reveal the child. The following key is used:

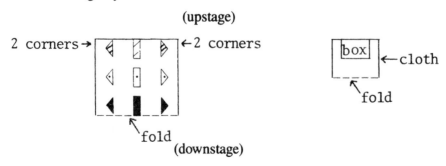

The bottom of the cloth (◀ ▮ ▶) is resting on the floor and is now a folded edge as the result of L's activity in the beginning of the second movement. (See page 143.) The fold is designated by ------. As the cloth is inverted, folded, etc., the various parts continue to be referred to by the original markings given in the key, i.e., ▶ of the cloth always refers to the corner which was ▶ just after the beginning of the second movement.

Illustration of Use of Key

(Second Movement)

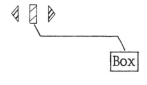

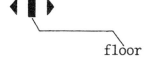

In the third movement the cloth is very deliberately folded and refolded as part of the dance. Additional use is made of the key. For example:

Resultant movement of the cloth - it ends in a side-side direction. (See page 205.)

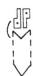

Cloth ends in a forward-backward direction after a resultant somersaulting action. (See page 207.)

In reconstructing the "folding" section of the dance, it is suggested that a cloth actually be marked with the key on both sides in order to keep track of the various corners. If the cloth is correctly folded and placed, it will unfold correctly at the end of the dance. To test the folding, have one person standing on the stage right side of the box take the top corner with the right hand and the fourth corner down with the left hand and have another person on the stage left side take the second corner from the top with the left hand and the third corner with the right hand. Pull the cloth, stretching it out. If this is accomplished without a twist in the material, the score has been worked out correctly, and the cloth folded properly.

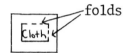

Aerial view of cloth on box
at the end of the "Folding"
section. (See page 207.)

Glossary

Timing

This movement score is often marked with 𝄴 . In general the dance is musically organized around the sound of the melodic line rather than the metric bar lines. There are few "counts"; much of the movement is performed on breath rhythms. The 𝄴 is used in this score to mean that the movement begins and ends where the ad lib begins and ends, but in between the movement is "fitted in"; where the various count marks and bar lines fall is only approximate and should not be interpreted literally.

One possible way of studying this score would be to read a section for movement, consult the marked music score to see where the movement occurs and then try to relate the two by listening to the music. The Dance Notation Bureau has available a marked music score, and it is strongly recommended that it be consulted.

Solid lines are musical bar lines; dotted bar lines are dance bars.

Please note that in the third movement the basic notation unit changes several times. The changes coincide with musical changes and are marked like this:

♩ = ▯   then later   ♩ = ♪ ; ♪ = ▯

Numbering System

```
        3)
        2)
  1    ①
  #     #
measure   counts
   dancer's
```

Floor Plans

The Box remains static throughout the dance. At the opening of the dance the entire cast is on stage in a tableau; since some of the dancers do not move from this position until much later in the dance, they are omitted from some of the early floor plans.

Notation Usages

J's movement, in general, is expansive. Unless otherwise indicated, his steps are assumed to be large.

Young Girl - movement never makes a picture. Impressionistic, vague, changing. Nothing is ever quite symmetrical. First sequence - a little frightened, like a squirrel or a rabbit. A light, air dance.

For all dancers - never "wind up." Move directly and simply from one point to another without any extraneous activity in the arms, legs or body. When no arm movement is indicated, do not allow the arms to flop around.

Day on Earth is a highly emotional dance. Throughout, the motivation is of greater consequence than the movement itself, the movement being merely the vessel for the emotional content. The whole body speaks, not just the face.

Although a realistic piece, the dance is also symbolic. Each character is an archetype, an ideal.

ꙇ	=	Just above the knee
ꙇ	=	Just below the knee
ꞓ	=	Just above the elbow
+.	=	Just below right hip joint - at very top of thigh
(breath symbol)	=	A breath (See page 140.)
(diminishing strength symbol)	=	Diminishing strength ending in passive weight
(place high symbol)	=	"In the place high area," i.e., more or less place high (See page 192.)
(black diamond symbol)	=	A black diamond placed within a direction symbol means gesture in an undeviating two-dimensional path with the direction judged according to the resultant (new) front. (See page 141.)

In this score there are moments when neither a ○ or ◇ is written for the arms during a torso tilt. The hold signs are deliberately omitted because the arms are not to be noticed, and the performer does not perform a clear ○ or ◇ , but something in between the two.

(symbol) = (symbol)   An easy, unforced turnout

    = Front of waist moves back and up. This movement pro-
duces a change in the shape of the body but is not a spacial
movement. It is equivalent to the former   , which is
now obsolete.

Note: Letitia Ide recalls Humphrey telling the dancers that her in-
spiration for the opening pose was a sculpture of Henry Moore. It
should have a sense of the monumental.

Regarding the Lament (page 189) she comments:

> *Mother is distracted with grief. She's off*
> *balance mentally. There is a lost quality*
> *to her movements, as she wavers back and*
> *forth from reality to memories.*

Another of her comments is that none of the dancers should ever
become sentimental. They are prototypical.

    = A "tick mark" placed on a cross of axes is the key used
to indicate that distal center analysis is being used to judge
direction for minor deviations. When judging the direction of a deviation with distal center analysis, the cross
of axes is located at the extremity of the moving part, and
the direction is judged from this cross of axes. Distal center
analysis may be indicated by the use of this key, or by
placing the tick directly on the appropriate direction pin.

Examples:

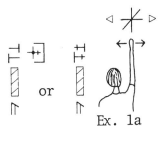

Ex. 1a

The right arm "waves" in a side to side action. We are not relating to side middle from the shoulder but rather to side as judged by a cross of axes located at the hand.

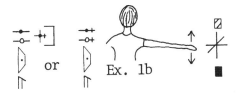

Ex. 1b

The right arm moves slightly "up and down," that is, slightly towards place high and place low, judged from a cross of axes centered on the extremity.

Note: *Without the tick on the deviation pin, proximal center analysis is used.* The cross of axes is centered on the point of attachment or fixed end of the moving part. The direction of the deviation can be thought of as "a small movement towards the next major direction."

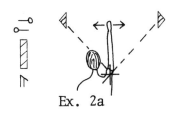

Ex. 2a

When a cross of axes is centered at the shoulder, the point of attachment, the arm moves a little towards right side high, and a little towards left side high.

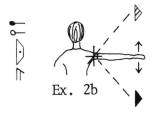

Ex. 2b

The arm moves a little towards right side high and a little towards right side low.

Examples 1a and 2a describe the *same* movement, with 1a using a distal center analysis (note the "tick marks" on the pins) and 2a using a proximal center analysis. Examples 1b and 2b also describe the same movement, with 1b using distal center analysis and 2b using proximal center analysis.

Alternate Version - L & J

Bars 163⁴ - 165

(See page 166)

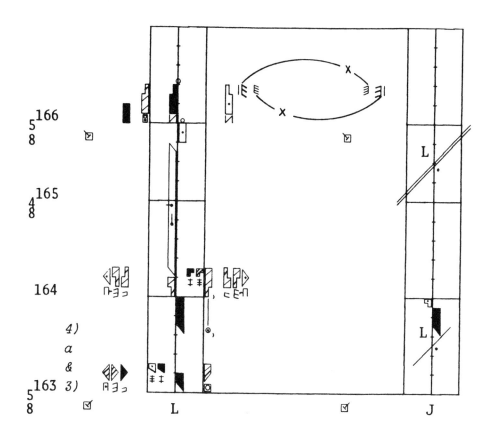

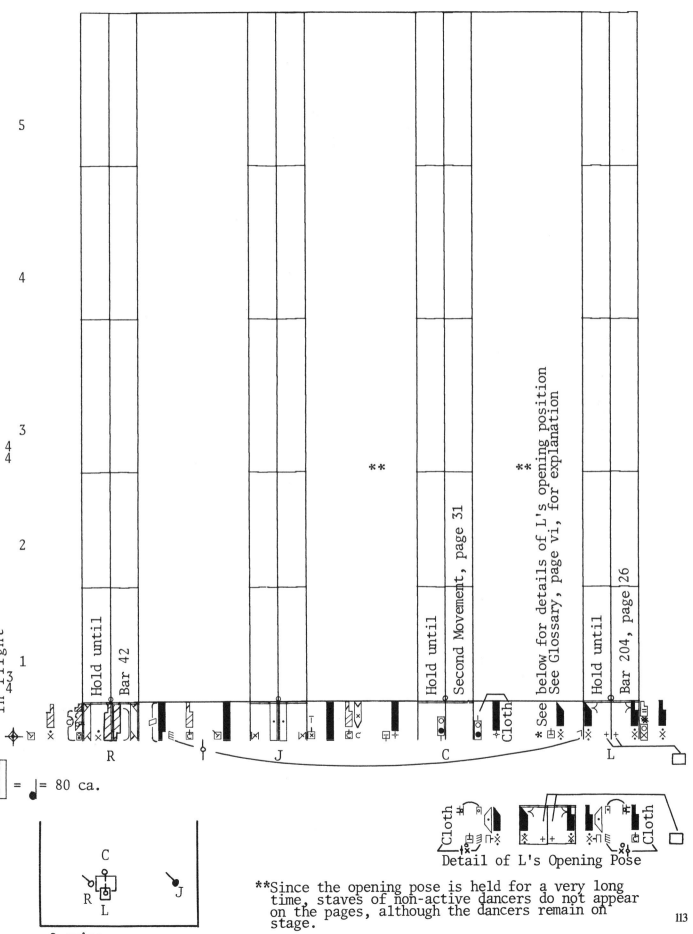

Detail of L's Opening Pose

**Since the opening pose is held for a very long time, staves of non-active dancers do not appear on the pages, although the dancers remain on stage.

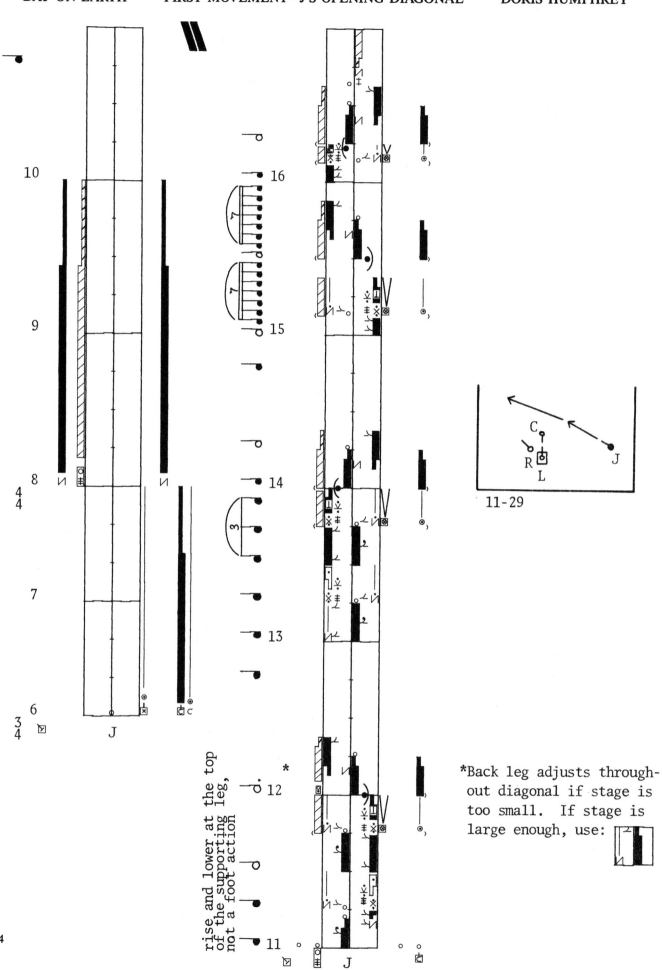

11-29

*Back leg adjusts through-
out diagonal if stage is
too small. If stage is
large enough, use:

rise and lower at the top
of the supporting leg,
not a foot action

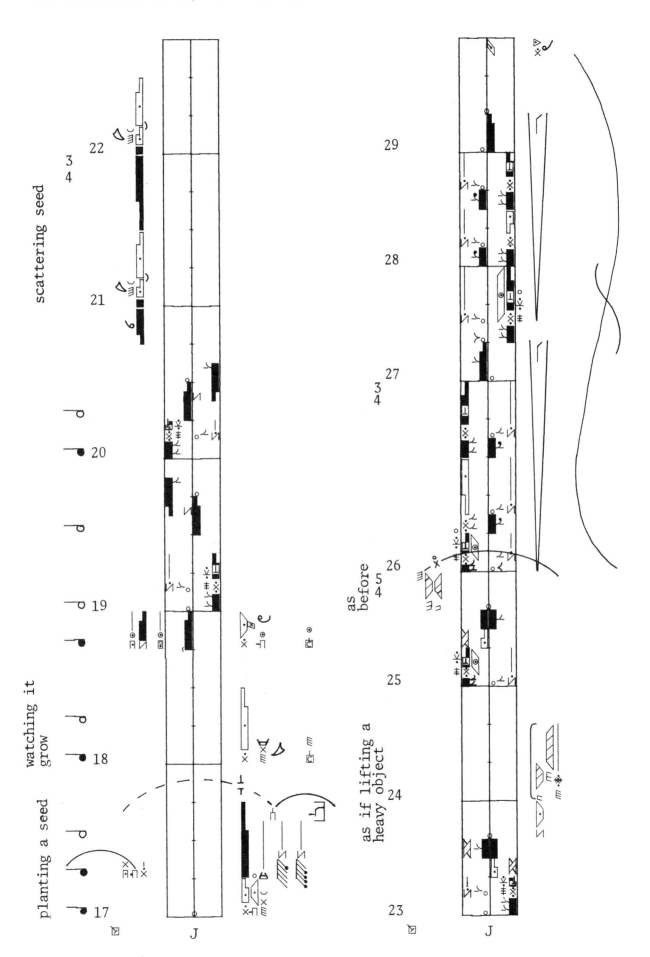

scattering seed

3
4

22

21

watching it
grow

planting a seed

20

19

18

17

J

29

28

3
4

27

as
before

5
4

26

25

as if lifting a
heavy object

24

23

J

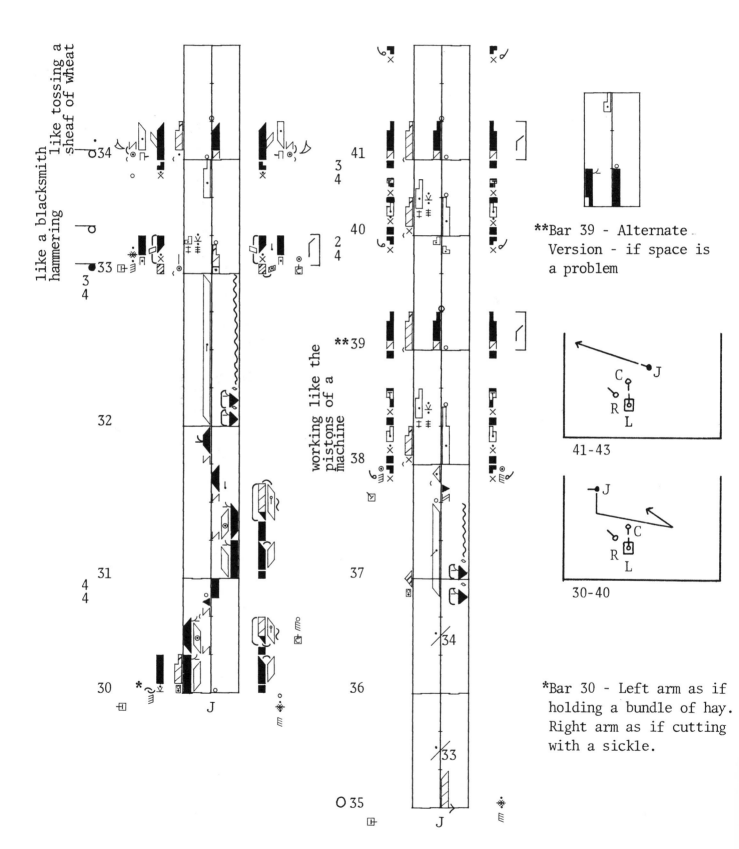

like tossing a
sheaf of wheat

like a blacksmith
hammering

working like the
pistons of a
machine

****Bar 39 - Alternate
Version - if space is
a problem**

41-43

30-40

***Bar 30 - Left arm as if
holding a bundle of hay.
Right arm as if cutting
with a sickle.**

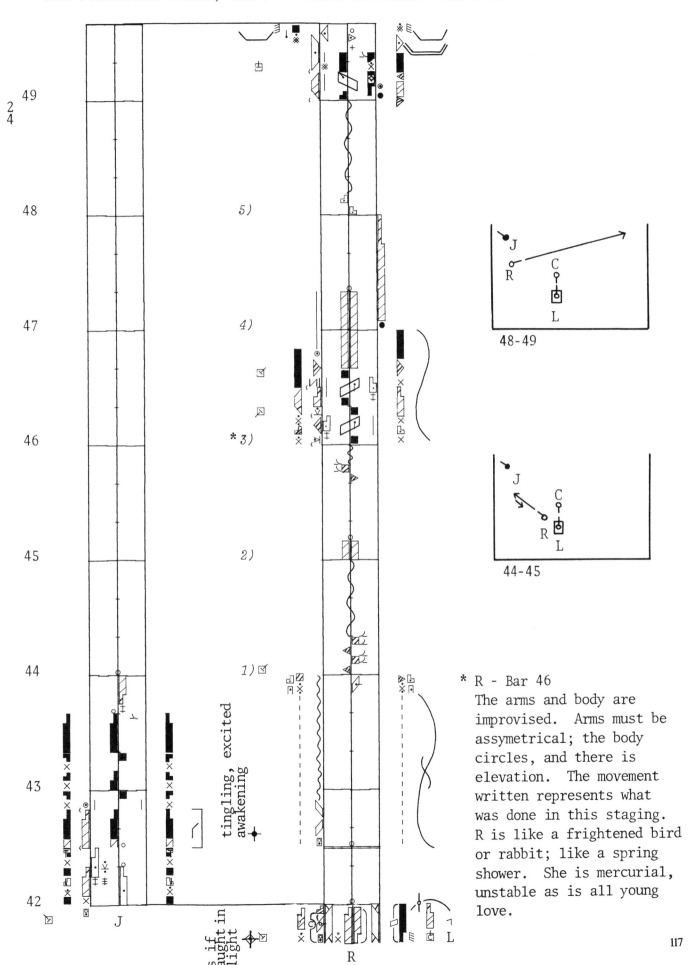

48-49

44-45

* R - Bar 46
The arms and body are
improvised. Arms must be
assymetrical; the body
circles, and there is
elevation. The movement
written represents what
was done in this staging.
R is like a frightened bird
or rabbit; like a spring
shower. She is mercurial,
unstable as is all young
love.

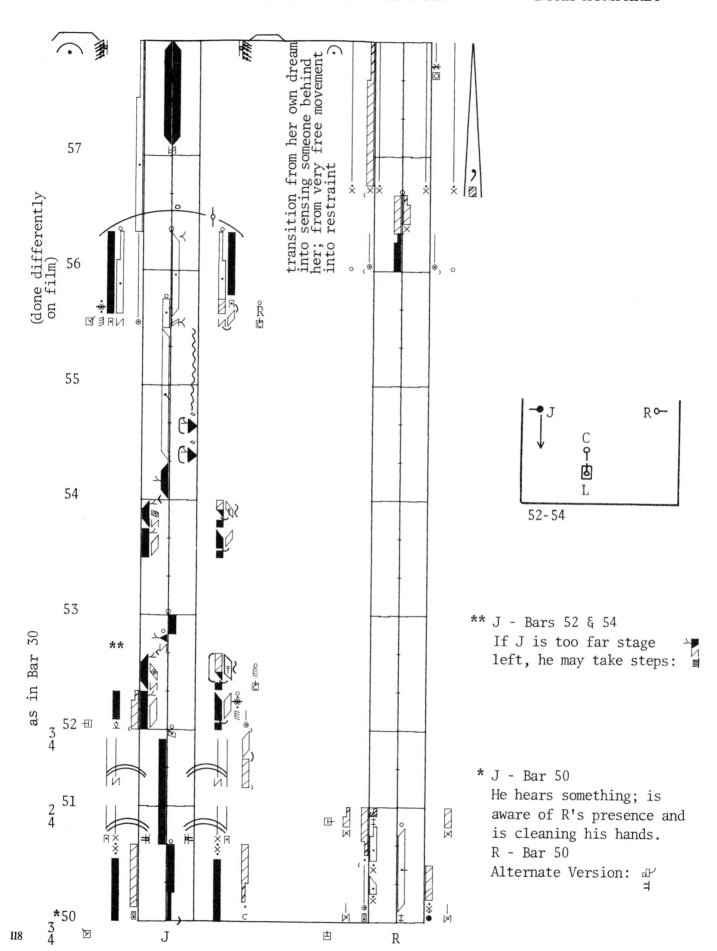

(done differently on film)

as in Bar 30

transition from her own dream into sensing someone behind her; from very free movement into restraint

57

56

55

54

53

52

51

50

3
4

2
4

3
4

J

R

52-54

** J - Bars 52 & 54
If J is too far stage
left, he may take steps:

* J - Bar 50
He hears something; is
aware of R's presence and
is cleaning his hands.
R - Bar 50
Alternate Version:

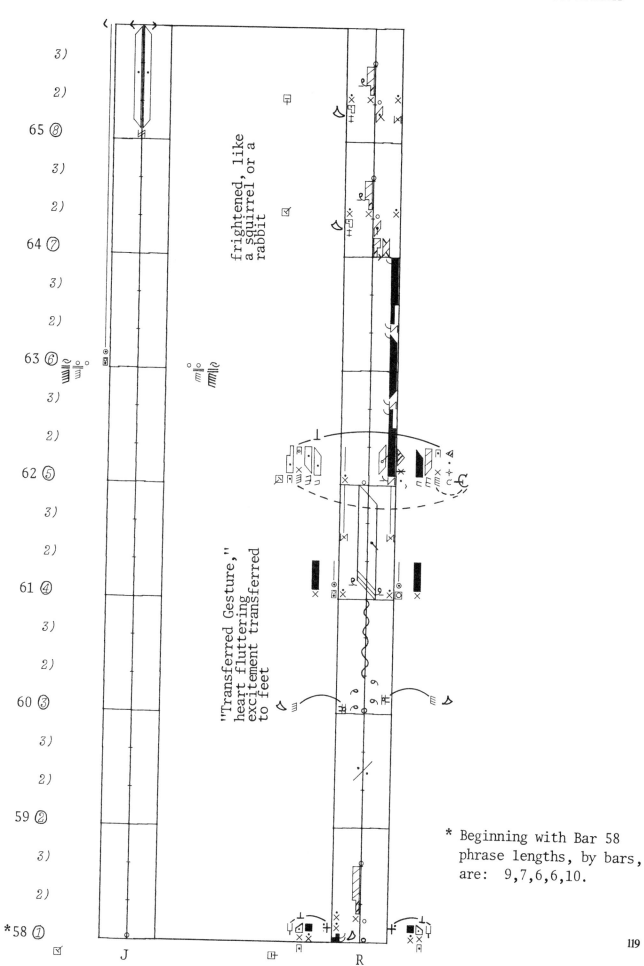

frightened, like
a squirrel or a
rabbit

"Transferred Gesture,"
heart fluttering
excitement transferred
to feet

3)

2)

65 ⑧

3)

2)

64 ⑦

3)

2)

63 ⑥

3)

2)

62 ⑤

3)

2)

61 ④

3)

2)

60 ③

3)

2)

59 ②

3)

2)

*58 ①

* Beginning with Bar 58
phrase lengths, by bars,
are: 9,7,6,6,10.

J

R

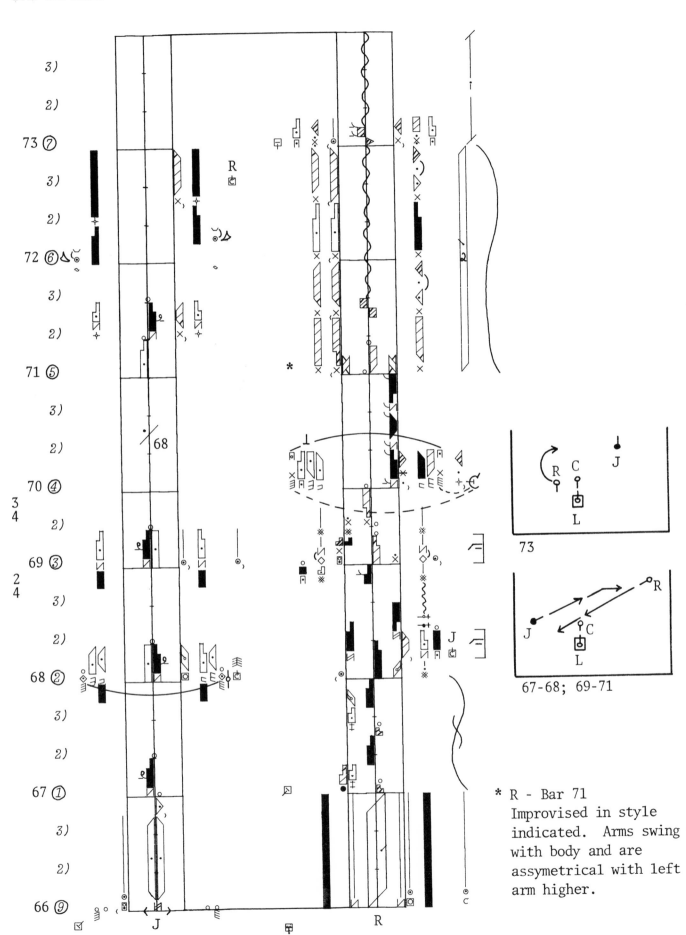

73

67-68; 69-71

* R - Bar 71
Improvised in style
indicated. Arms swing
with body and are
assymetrical with left
arm higher.

question and answer section

3)

2)

81 ②

3)

2)

80 ① *

3)

2)

79 ⑥

3)

2)

78 ⑤

3)

2)

77 ④

3)

2)

76 ③

3)

2)

75 ②

3)

2)

74 ①

J   凸   R   J

improvise as
before

playful

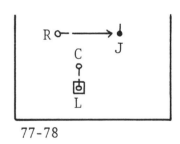

77-78

* J - Bars $80-81_1$ & $84-85_1$
On film:

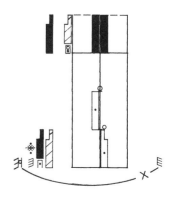

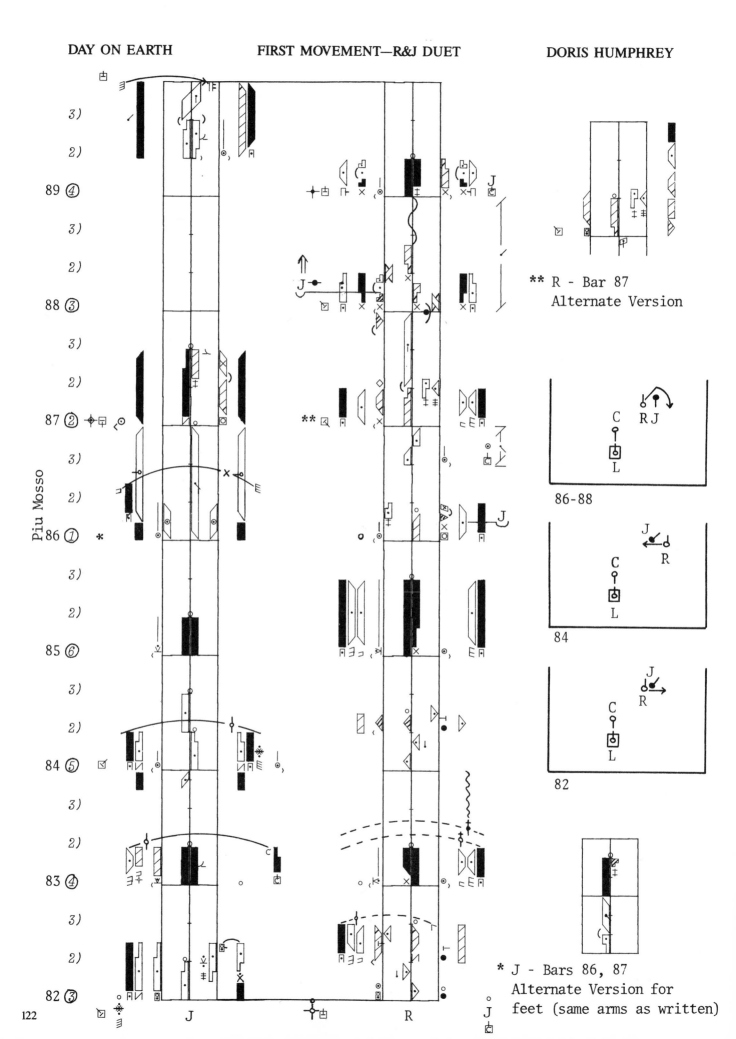

** R - Bar 87
Alternate Version

86-88

84

82

* J - Bars 86, 87
Alternate Version for
feet (same arms as written)

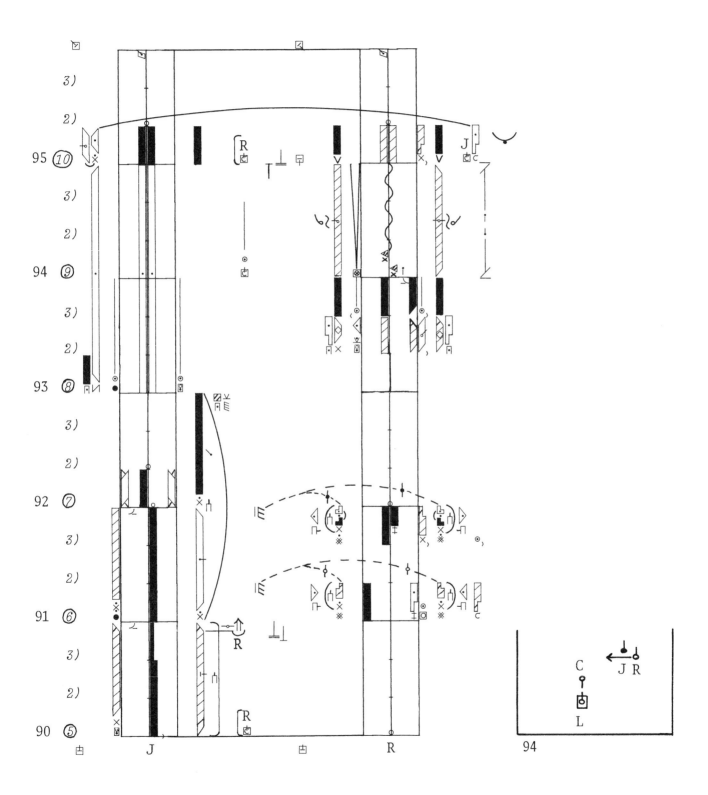

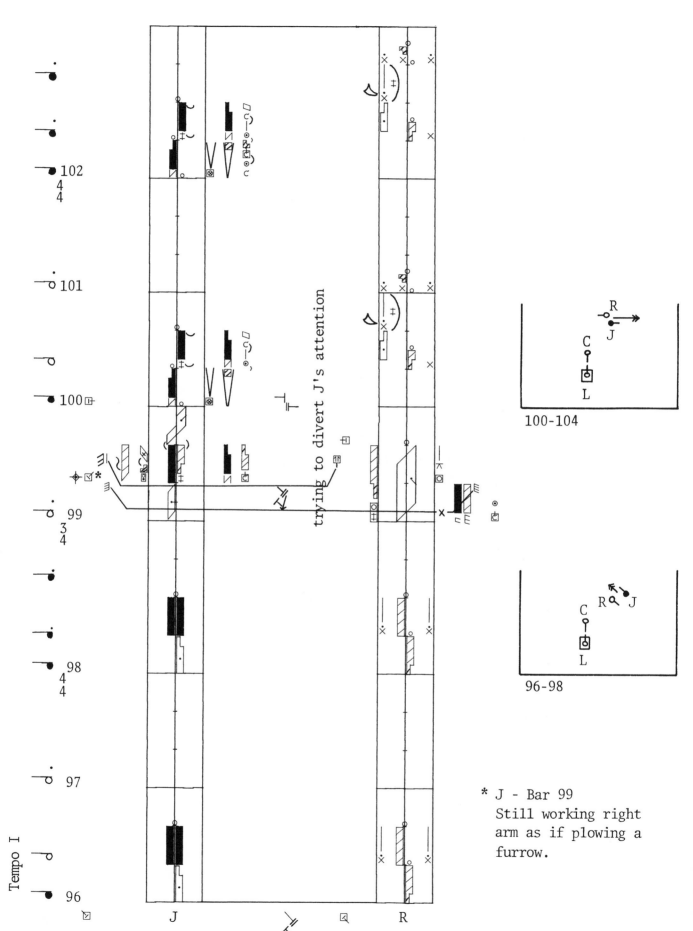

trying to divert J's attention

100-104

96-98

* J - Bar 99
Still working right
arm as if plowing a
furrow.

Tempo I

J   R

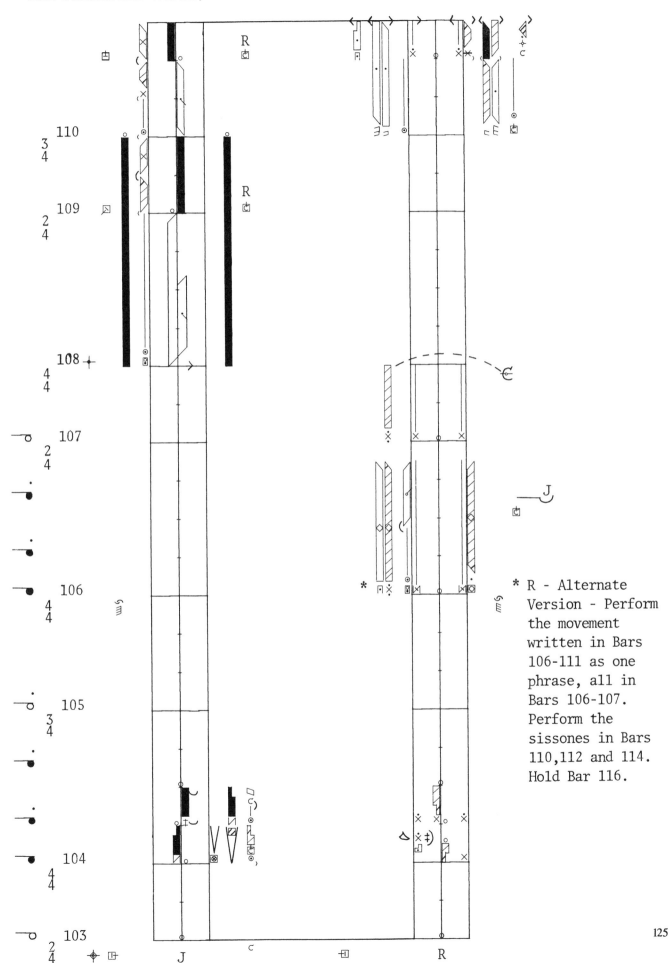

* R - Alternate
Version - Perform
the movement
written in Bars
106-111 as one
phrase, all in
Bars 106-107.
Perform the
sissones in Bars
110,112 and 114.
Hold Bar 116.

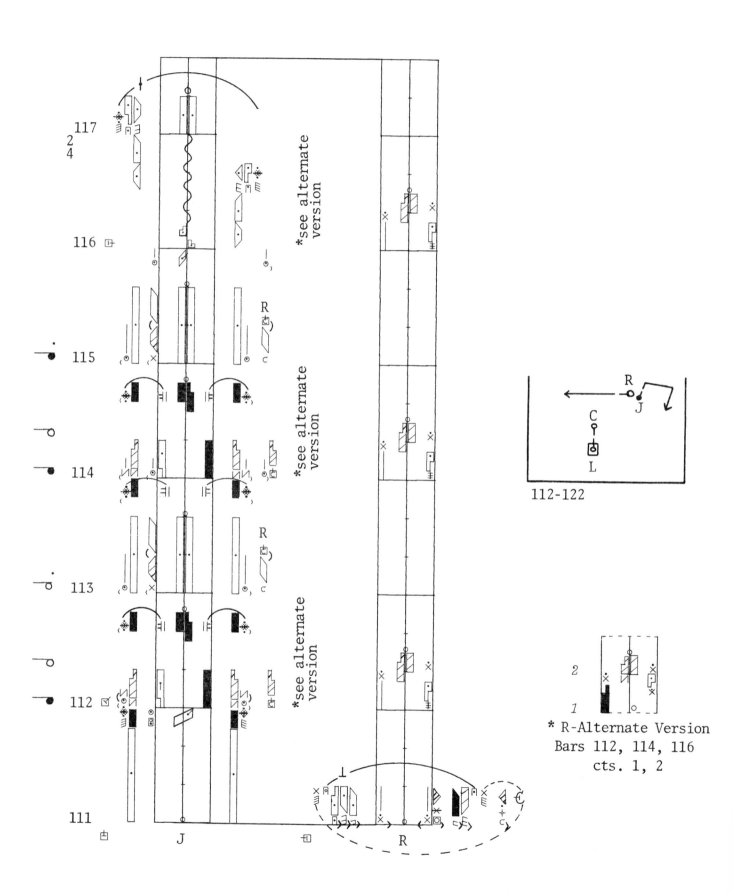

*see alternate version

*see alternate version

*see alternate version

112-122

2

1

* R-Alternate Version
Bars 112, 114, 116
   cts. 1, 2

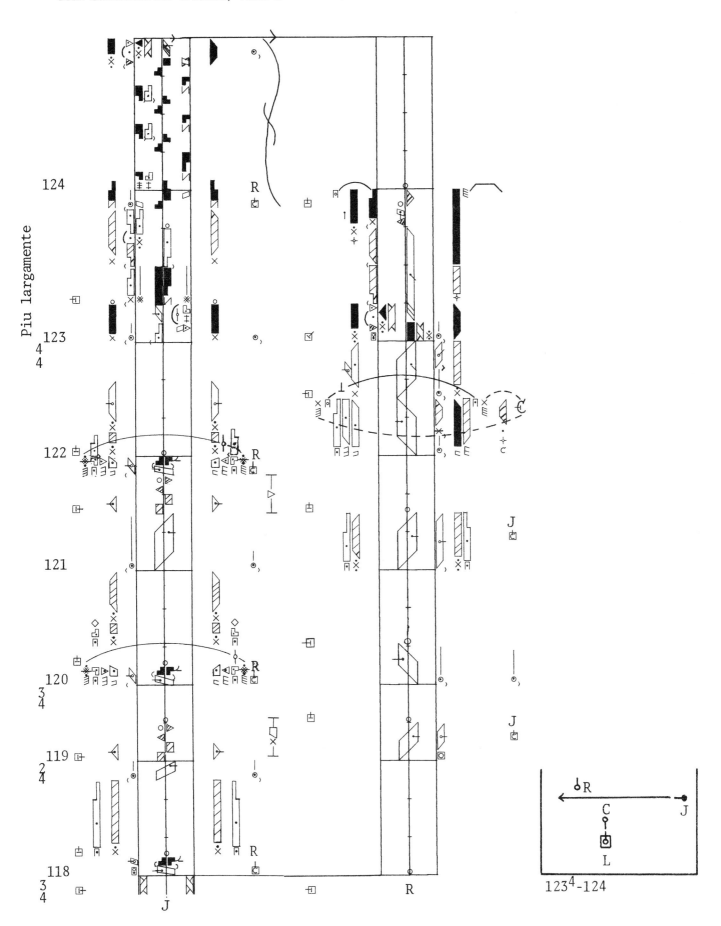

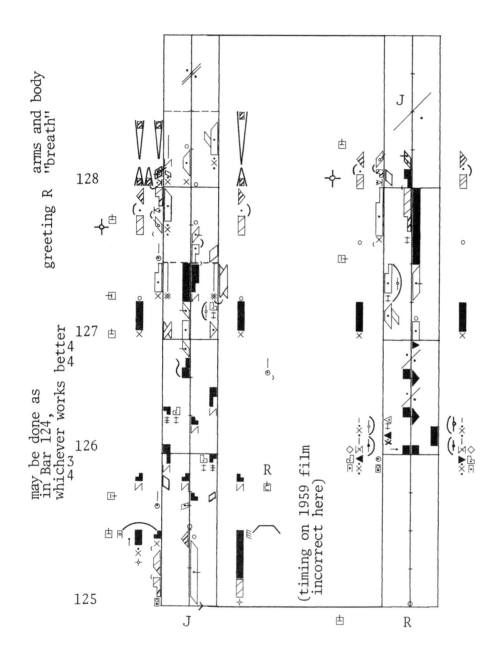

arms and body
greeting R "breath"

128

127

may be done as
in Bar 124,
whichever works better

126

(timing on 1959 film
incorrect here)

R

125

J   R

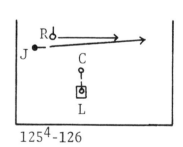

125⁴-126

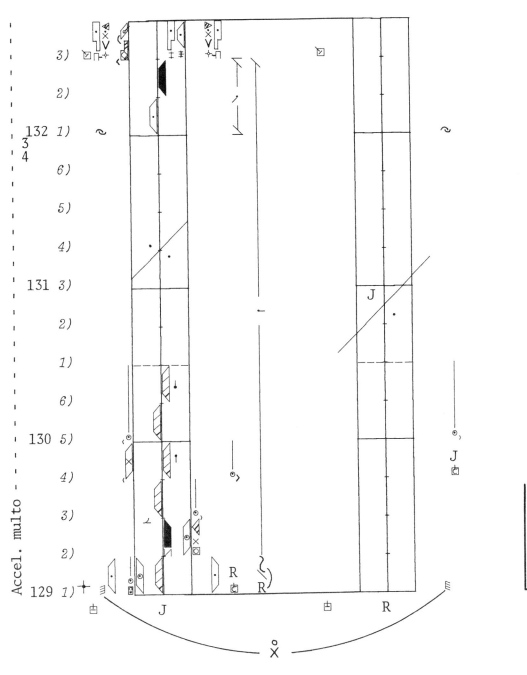

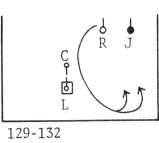

129-132

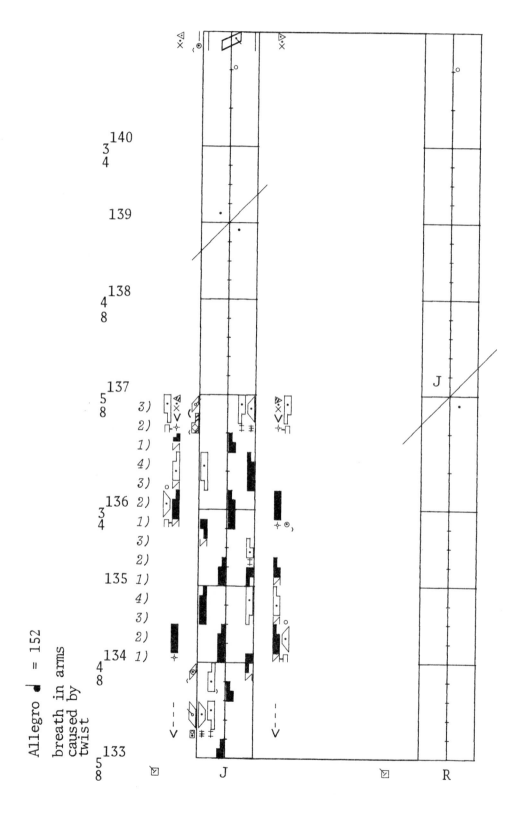

Allegro ♩ = 152

breath in arms
caused by
twist

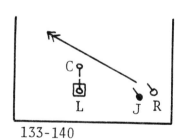

133-140

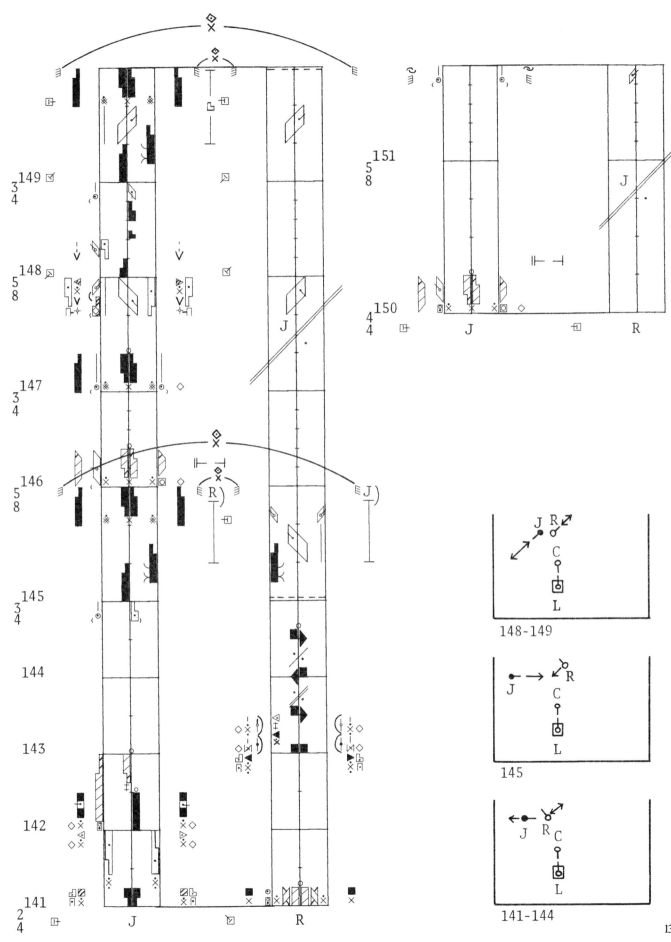

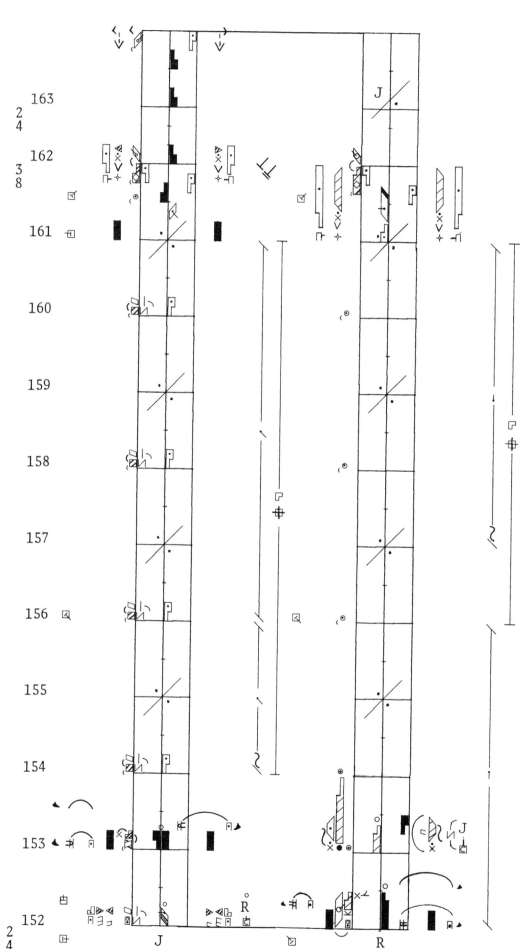

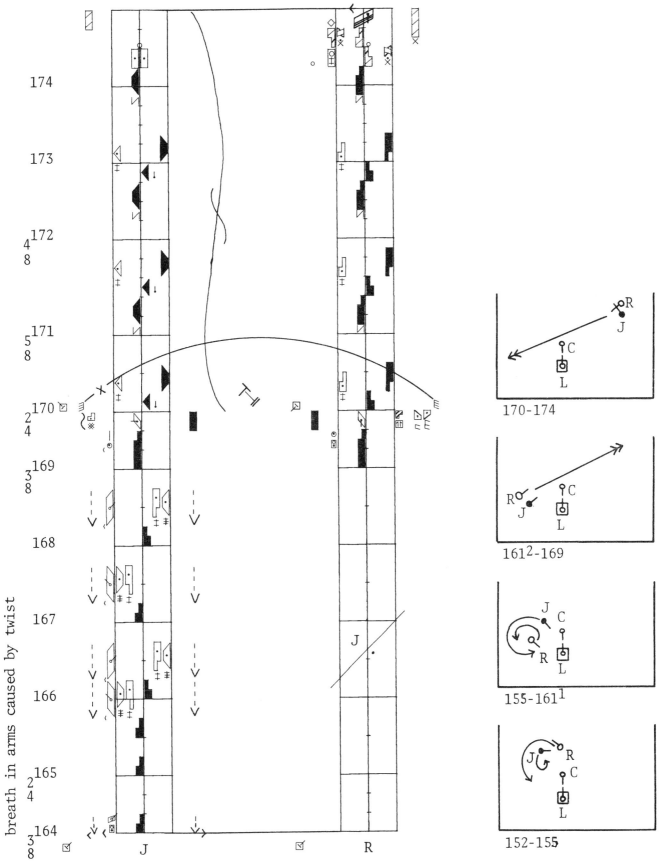

breath in arms caused by twist

170-174

161²-169

155-161¹

152-155

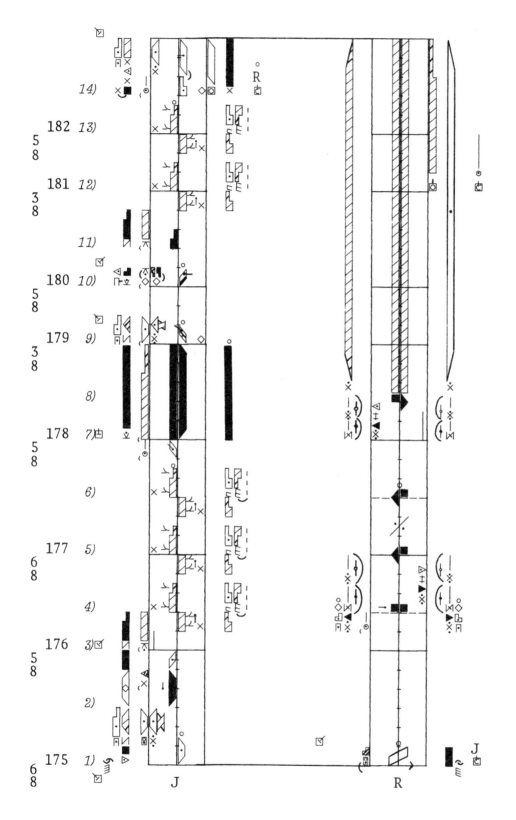

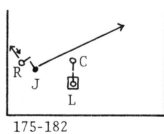

175-182

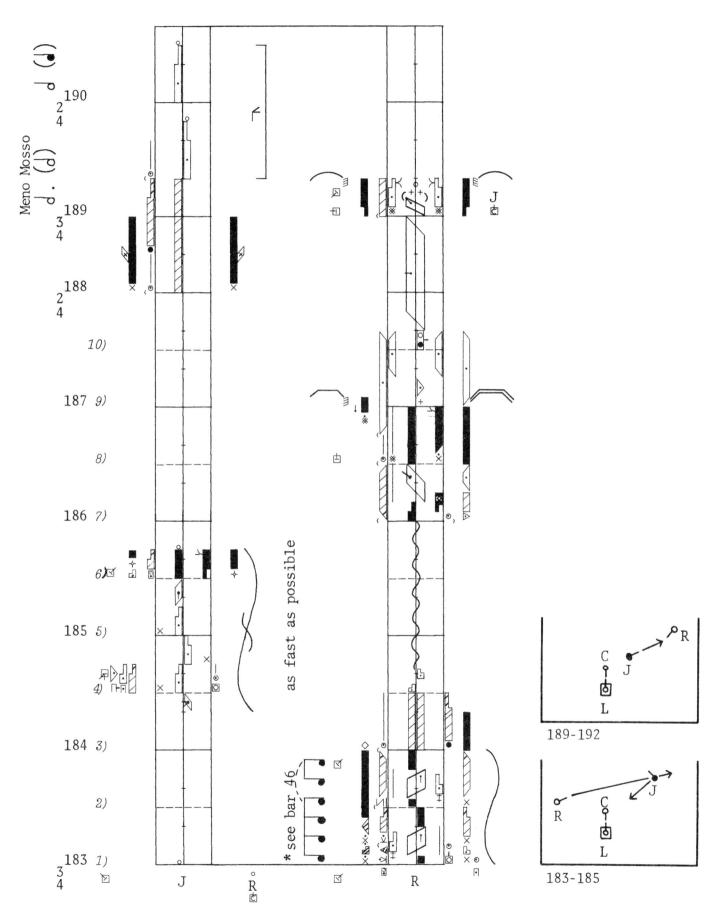

as fast as possible

* see bar 46

189-192

183-185

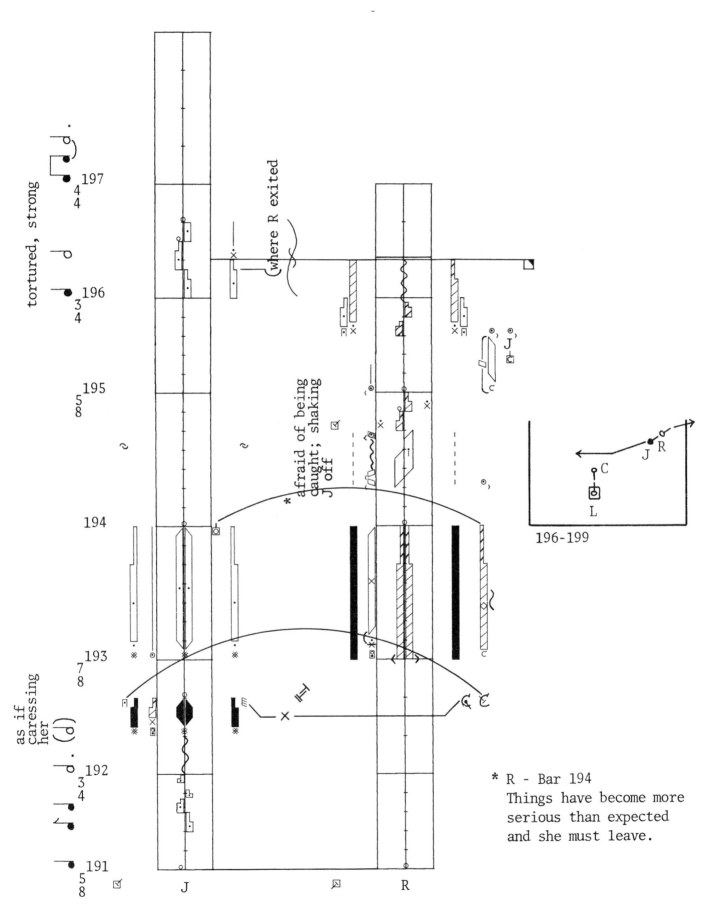

tortured, strong

197

196

195

194

193

192

191

as if
caressing
her

(where R exited)

* afraid of being
caught; shaking
J off

J

R

196-199

* R - Bar 194
Things have become more
serious than expected
and she must leave.

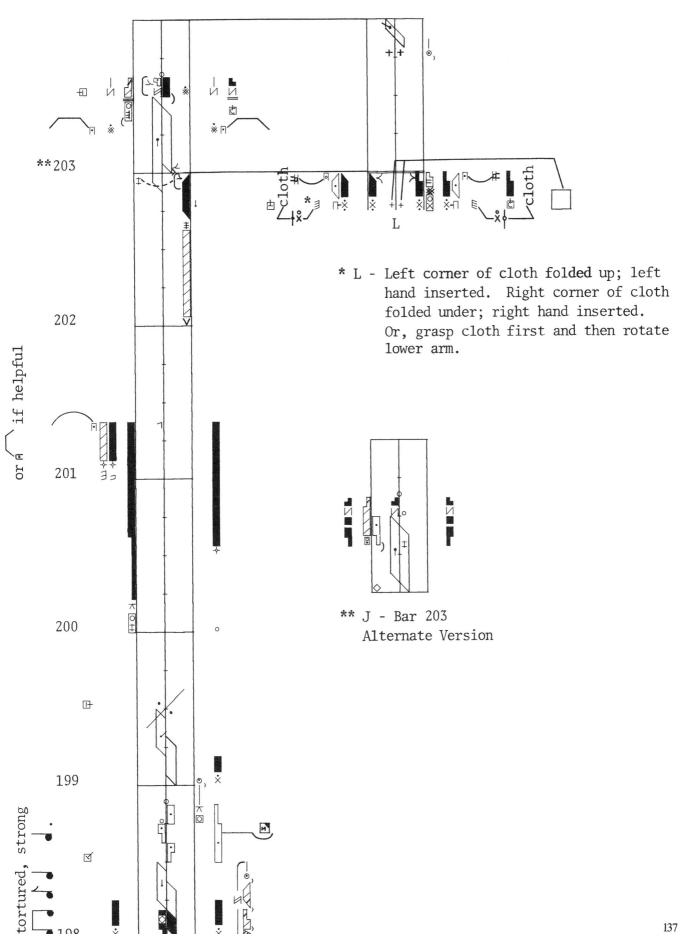

**203

cloth   cloth

L

* L - Left corner of cloth folded up; left
  hand inserted. Right corner of cloth
  folded under; right hand inserted.
  Or, grasp cloth first and then rotate
  lower arm.

202

or ‖ if helpful

201

** J - Bar 203
   Alternate Version

200

199

tortured, strong

198

J   C

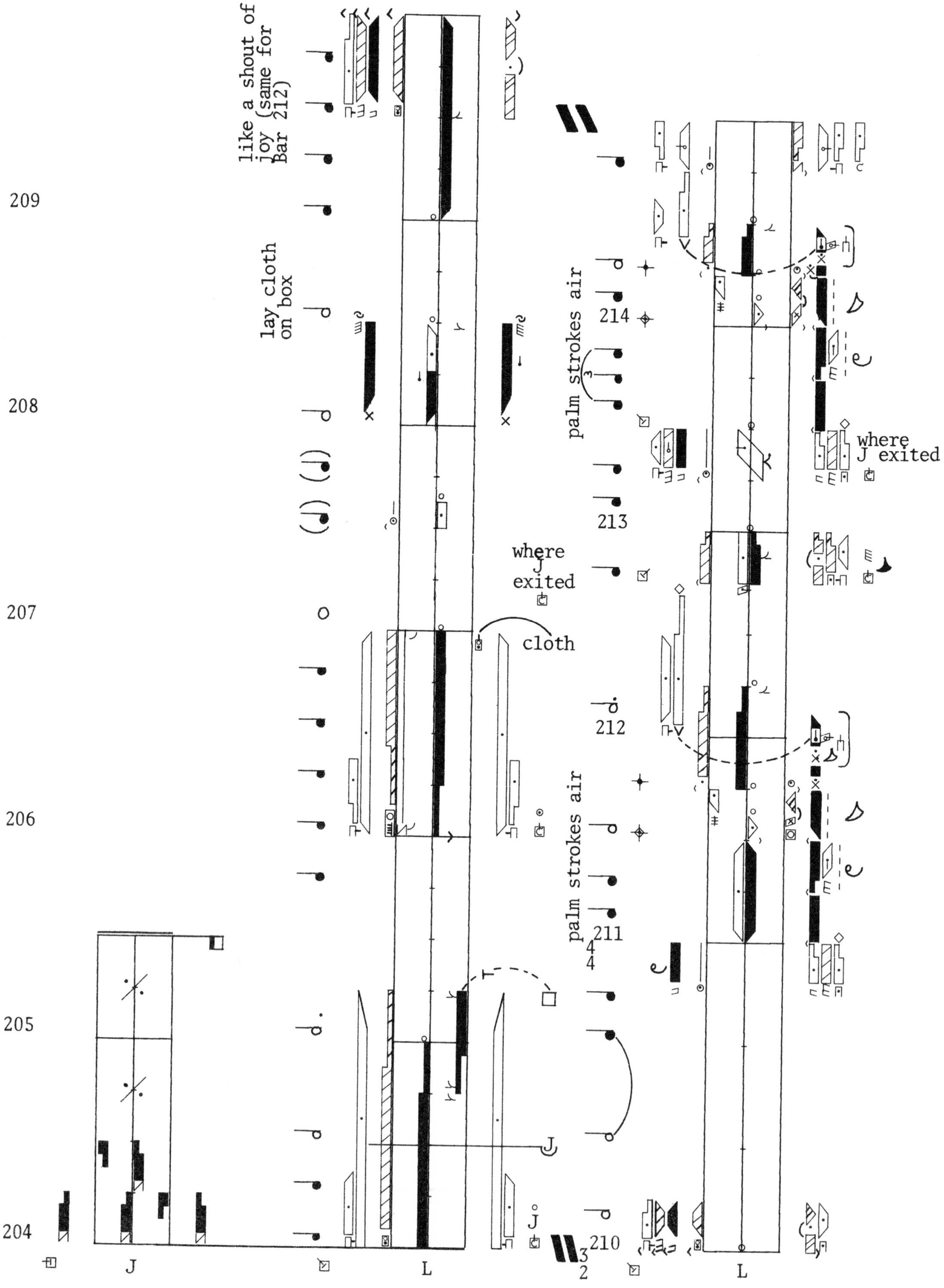

like a shout of
joy (same for
Bar 212)

lay cloth
on box

209

palm strokes air

214

208

where
J exited

where
J
exited

213

207

cloth

212

206

palm strokes air

211

205

J

204   J   210   L

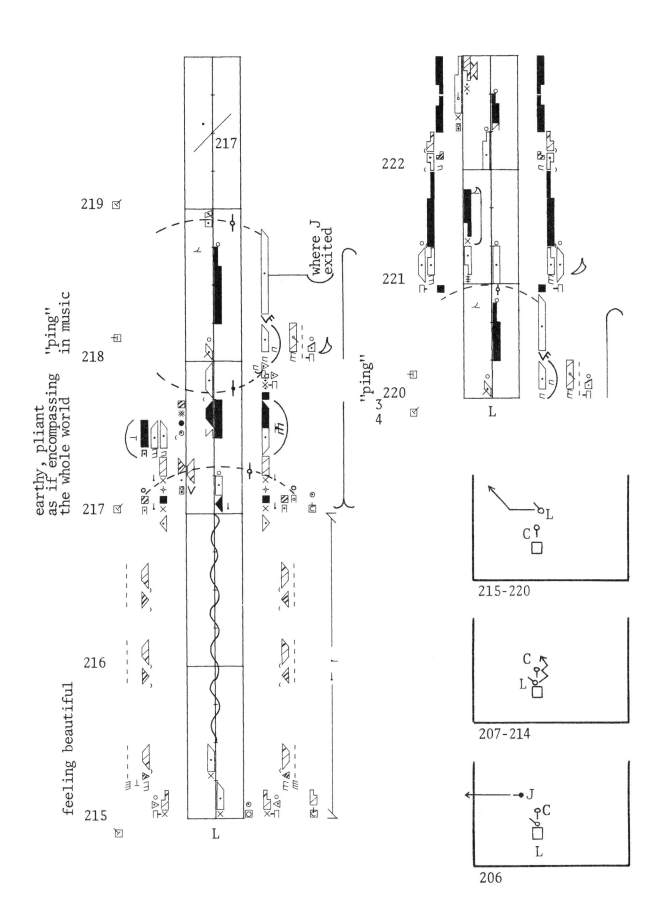

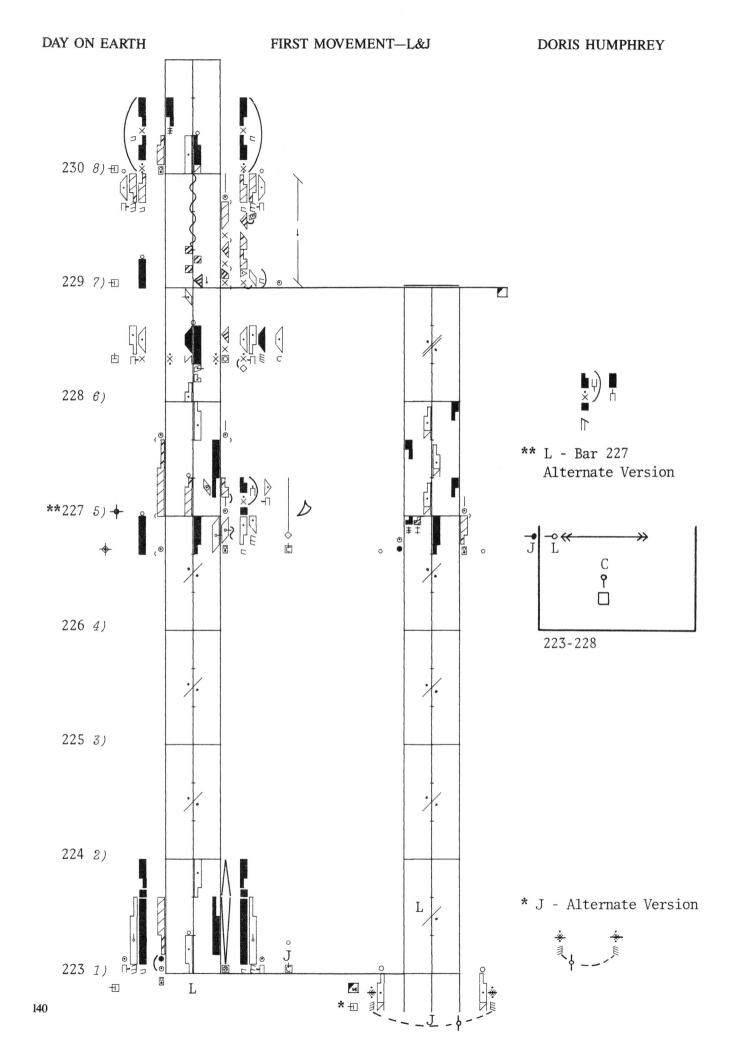

** L - Bar 227
Alternate Version

223-228

* J - Alternate Version

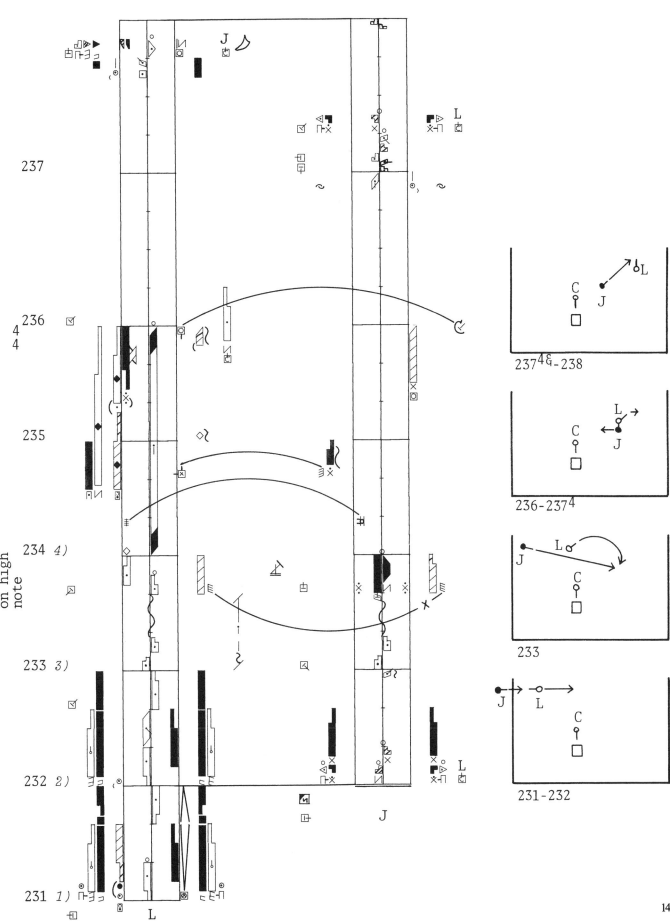

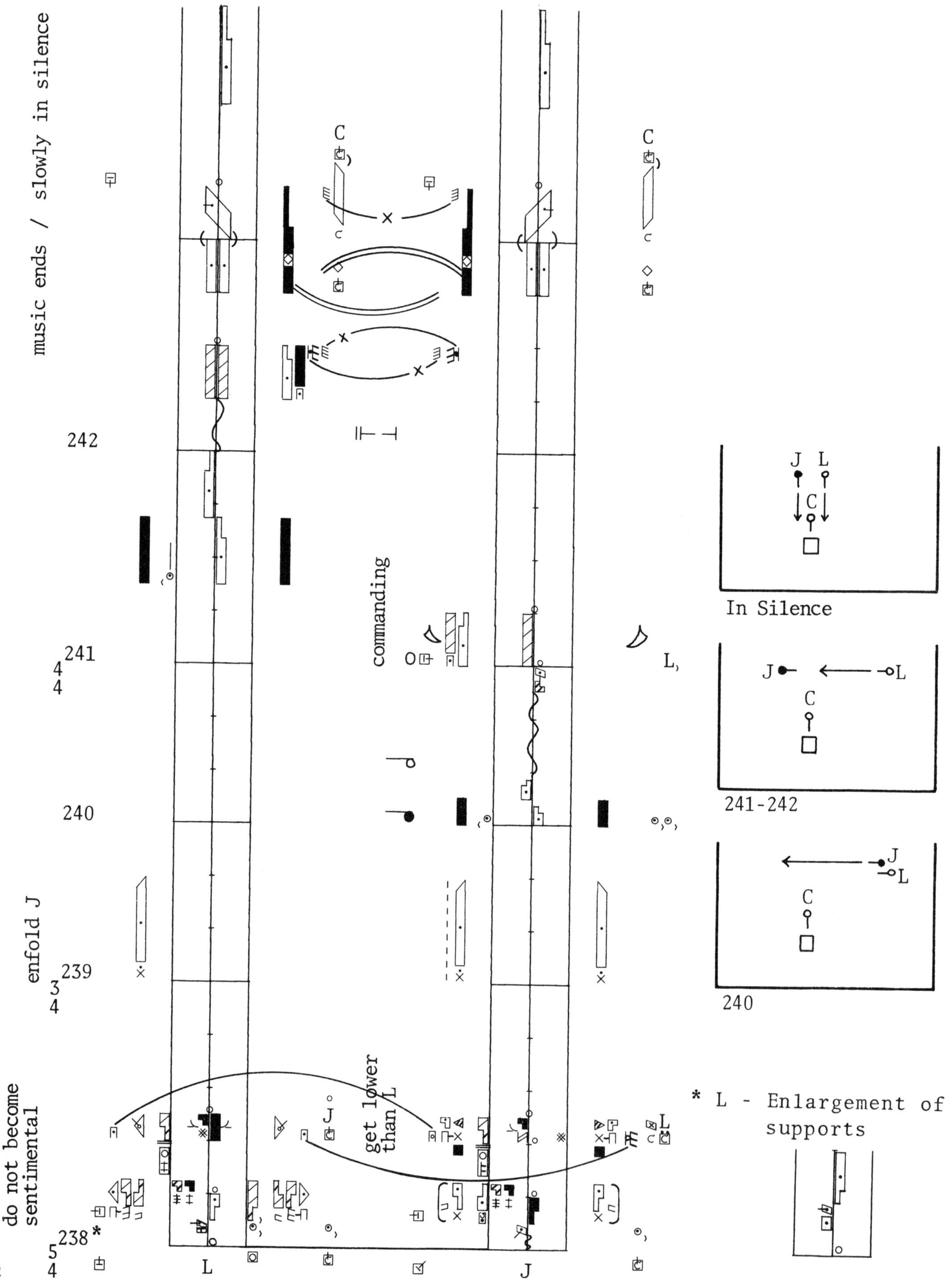

music ends / slowly in silence

commanding

242

241

240

enfold J

239

do not become sentimental

238 *

142

L

J

C

C

In Silence

241-242

240

* L - Enlargement of supports

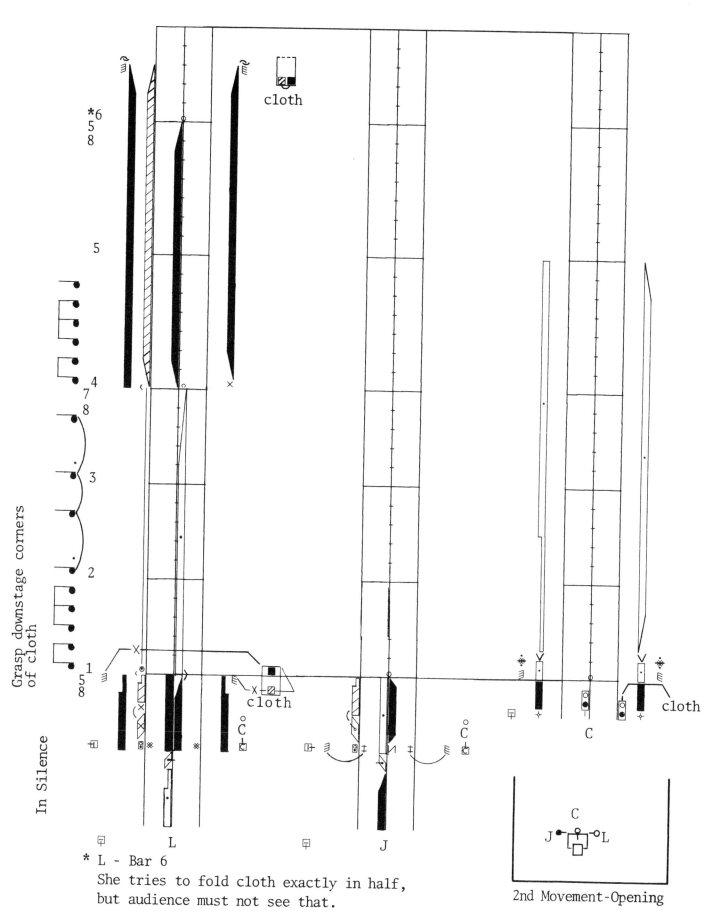

cloth

cloth

cloth

Grasp downstage corners of cloth

In Silence

L

J

C

2nd Movement-Opening

* L - Bar 6
She tries to fold cloth exactly in half,
but audience must not see that.

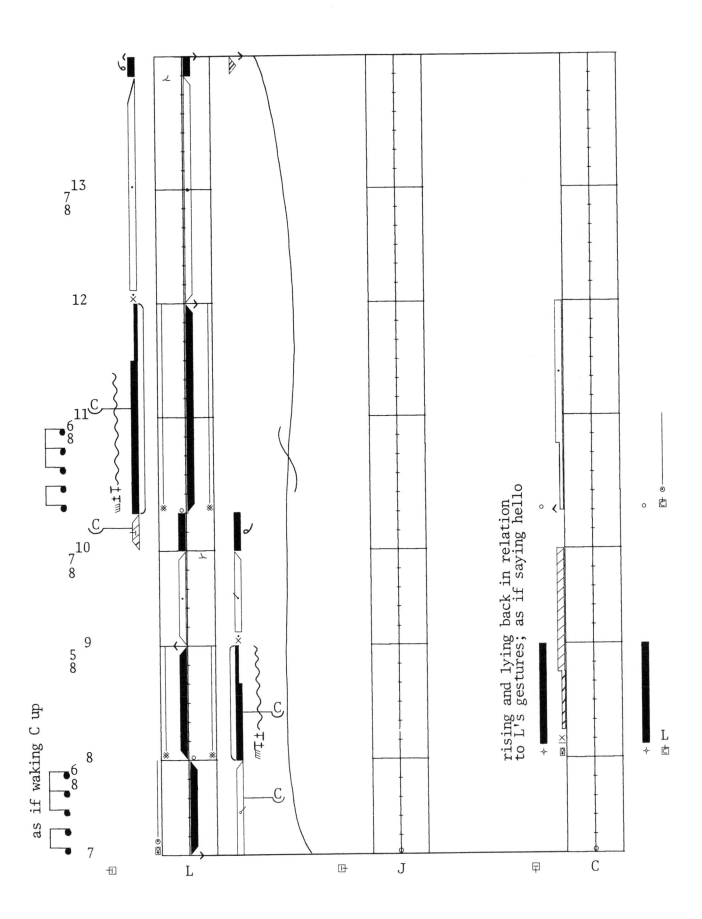

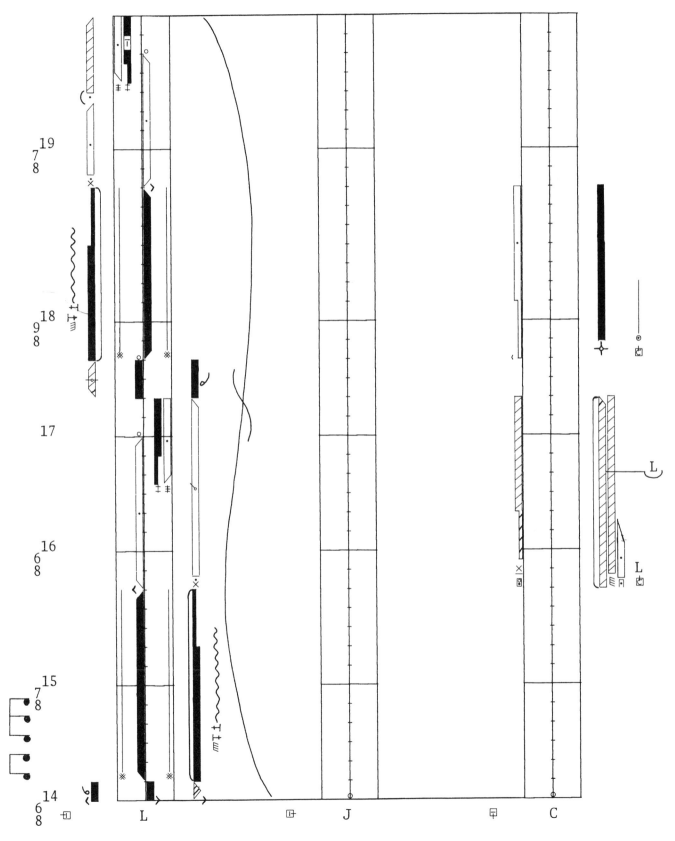

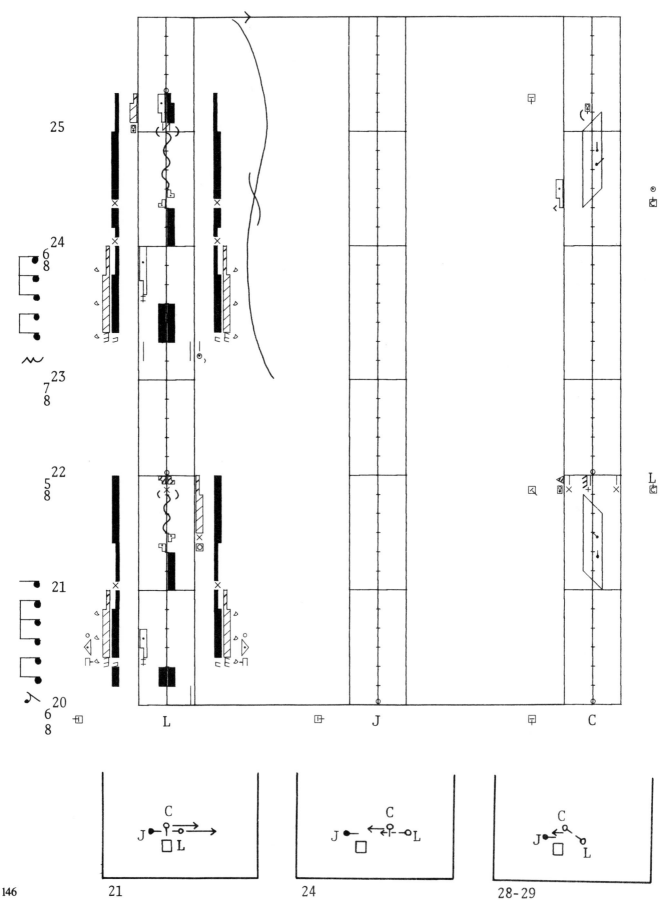

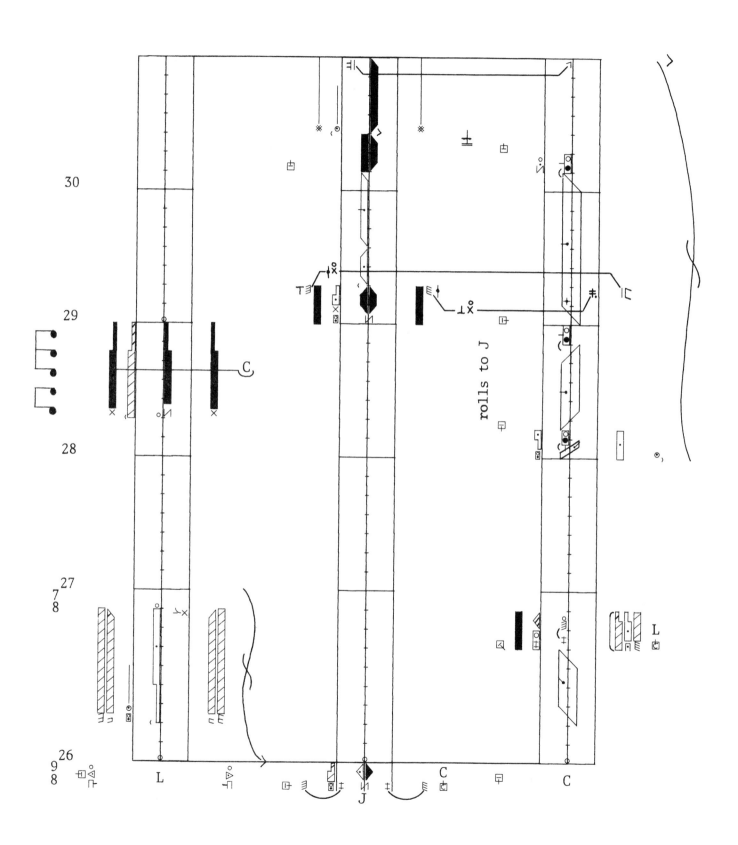

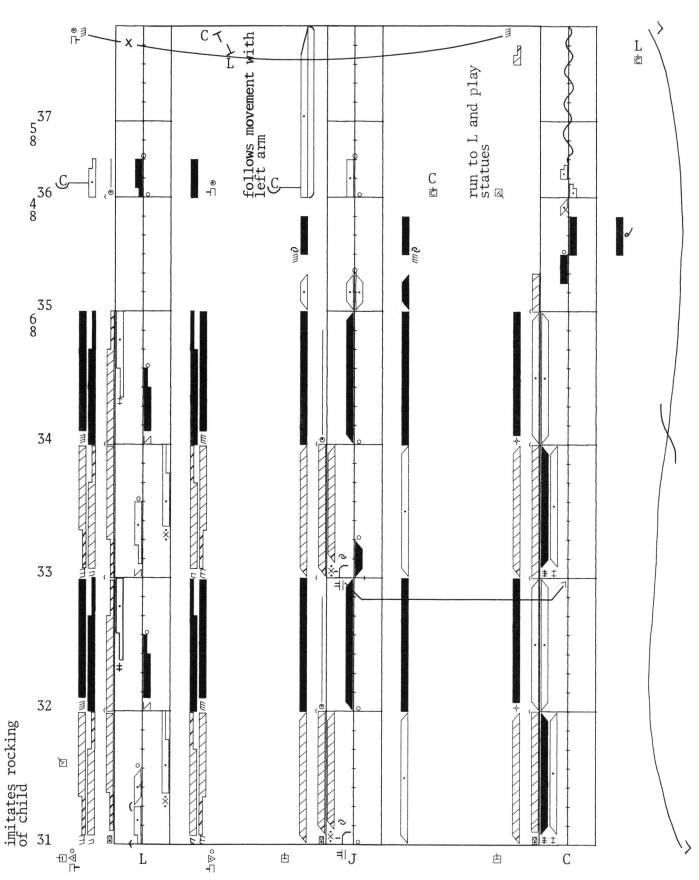

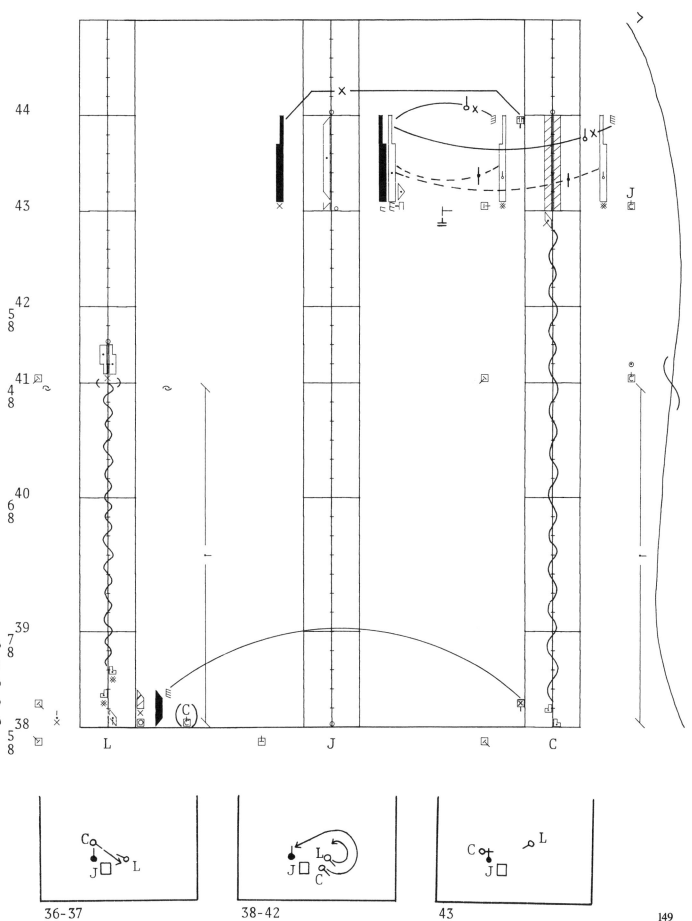

a gesture of admiration, great pride and love

53

52

C

C

51

50

49

48
5
8

47
3
8

46
4
8

45

L   J   C

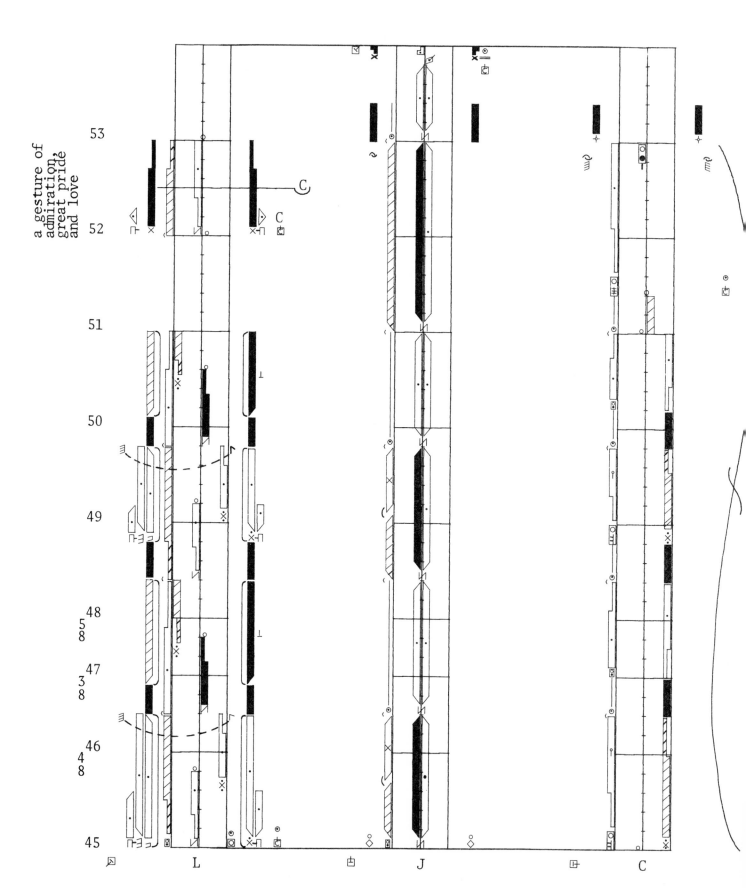

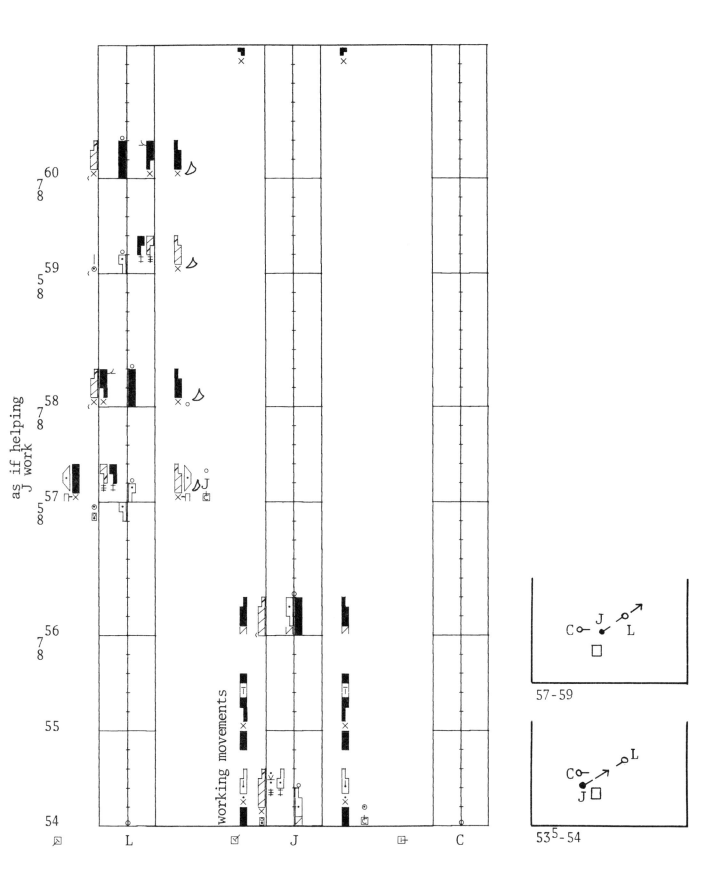

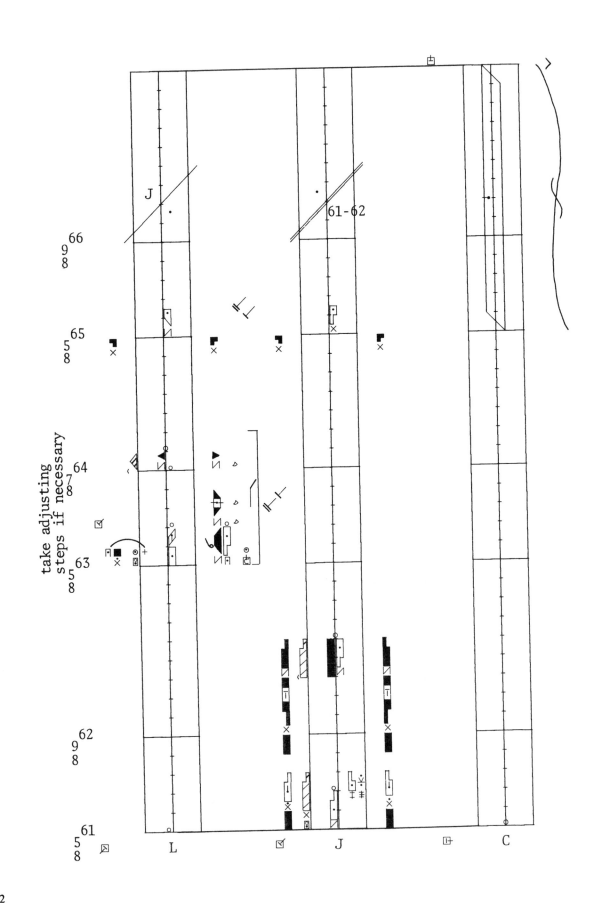

take adjusting
steps if necessary

61-62

J

66
9
8

65
5
8

64
7
8

63
5
8

62
9
8

61
5
8

L   J   C

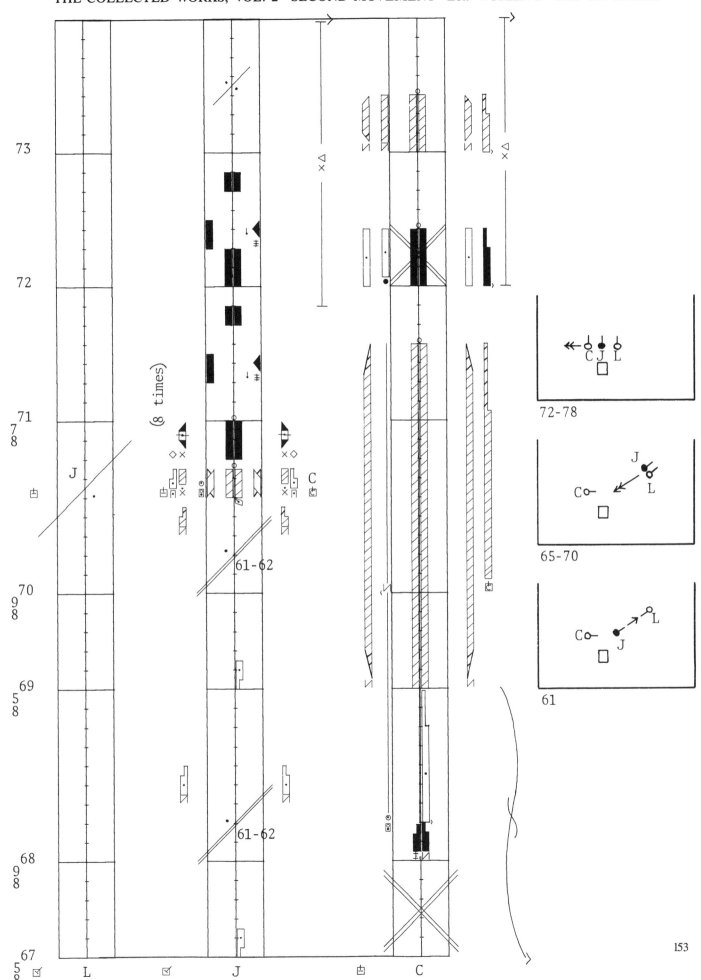

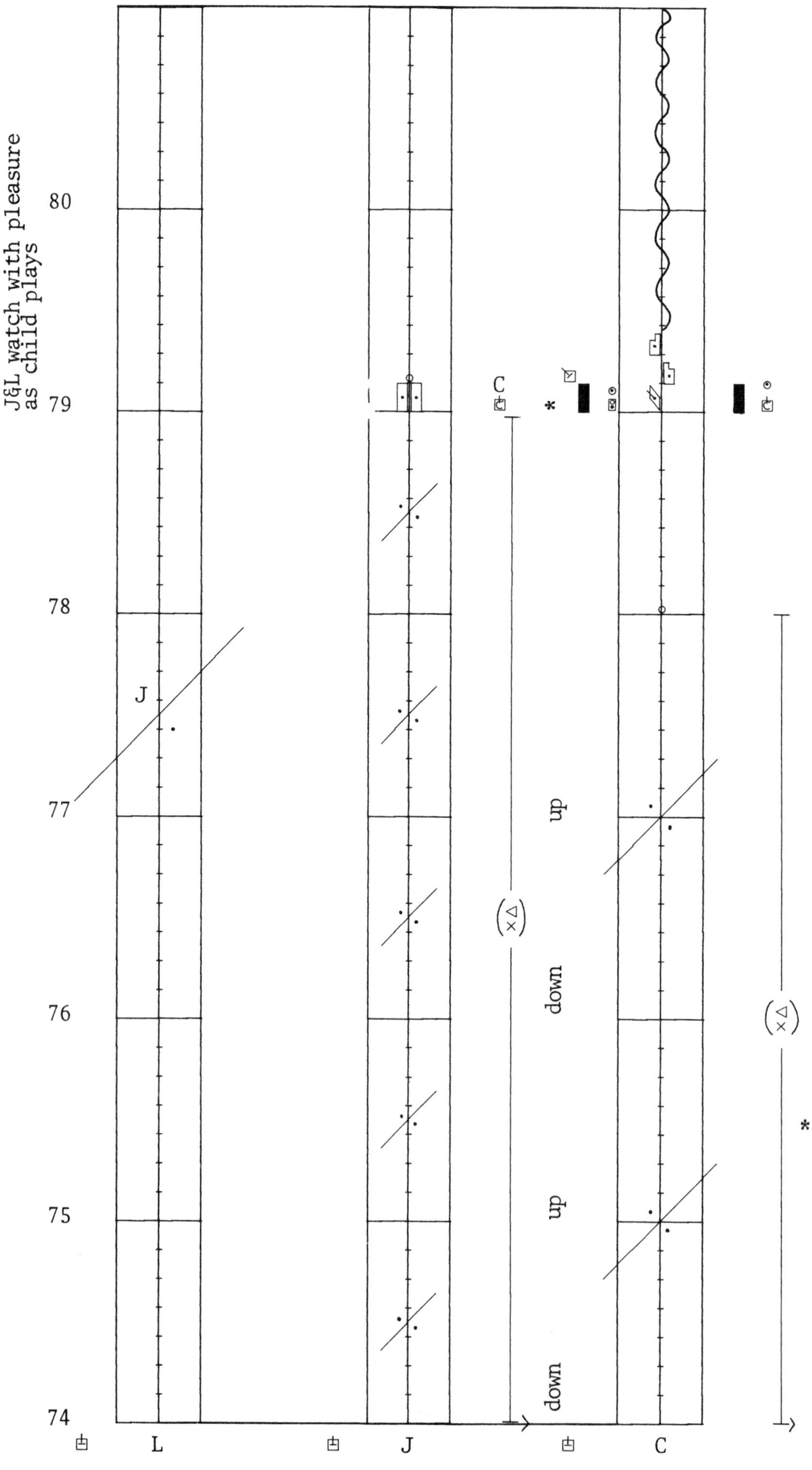

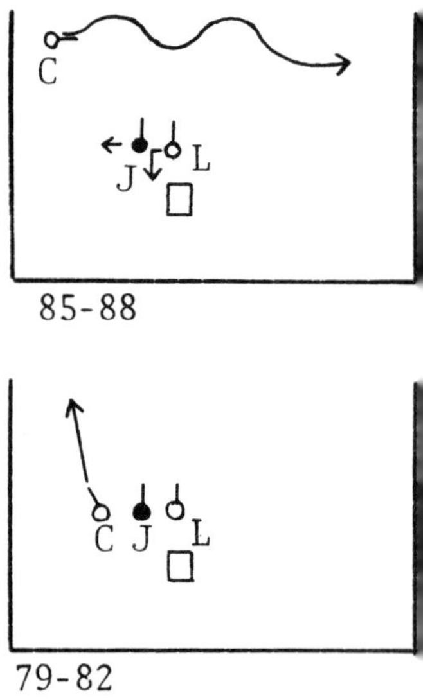

J&L watch with pleasure
as child plays

80

79

C

*

78

J

77

up

down

76

75

up

down

74

154

L   J   C

85-88

79-82

* C - Bar 79
All the movement in
the child's solo is
written as a guide,
as the solo is
taught in a general
way and fitted to
the movement capacity
of the child.

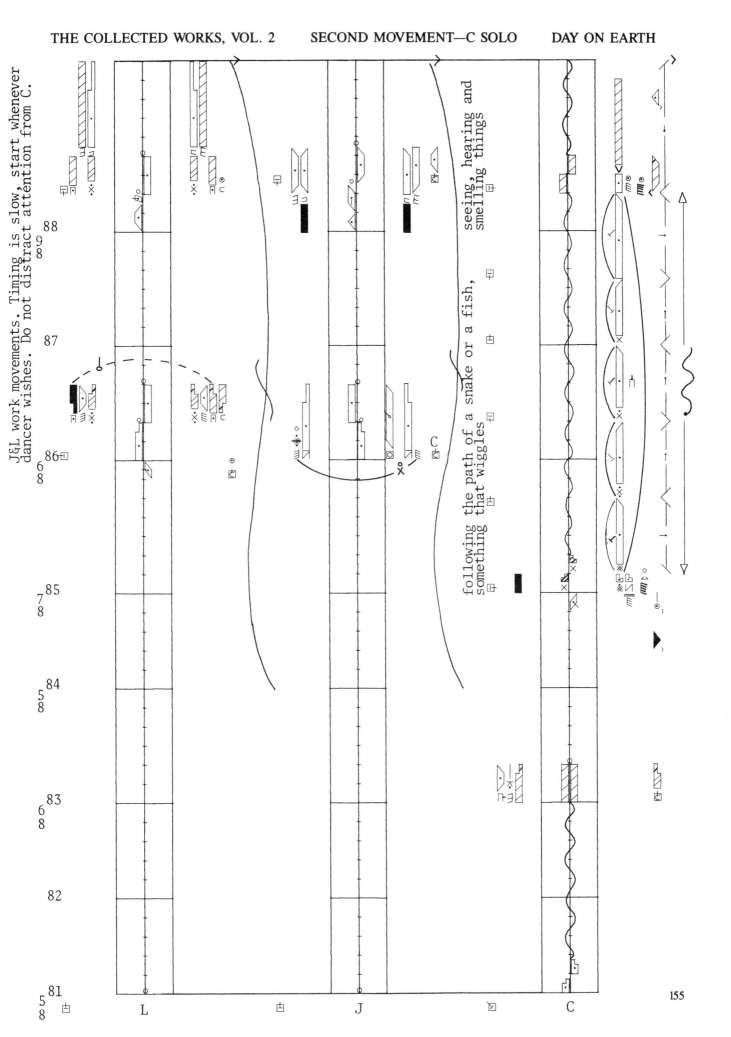

J&L work movements. Timing is slow, start whenever dancer wishes. Do not distract attention from C.

seeing, hearing and smelling things

following the path of a snake or a fish, something that wiggles

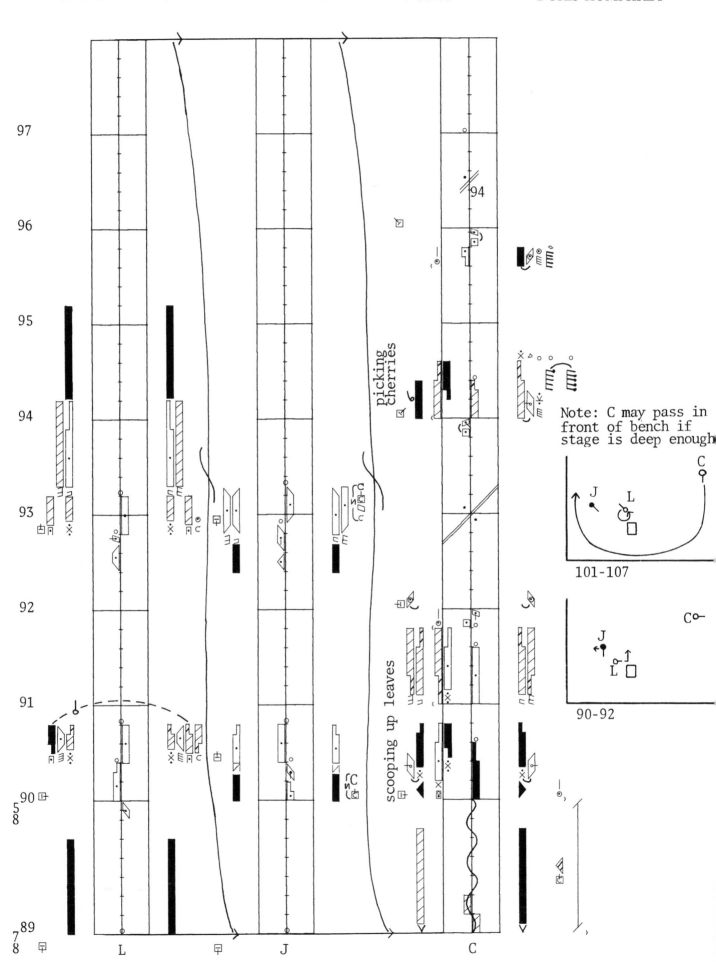

Note: C may pass in front of bench if stage is deep enough

101-107

90-92

picking cherries

scooping up leaves

J&L must perform these and the following movements related in time to one another, although the relationship, in time, to the music is somewhat ad lib.

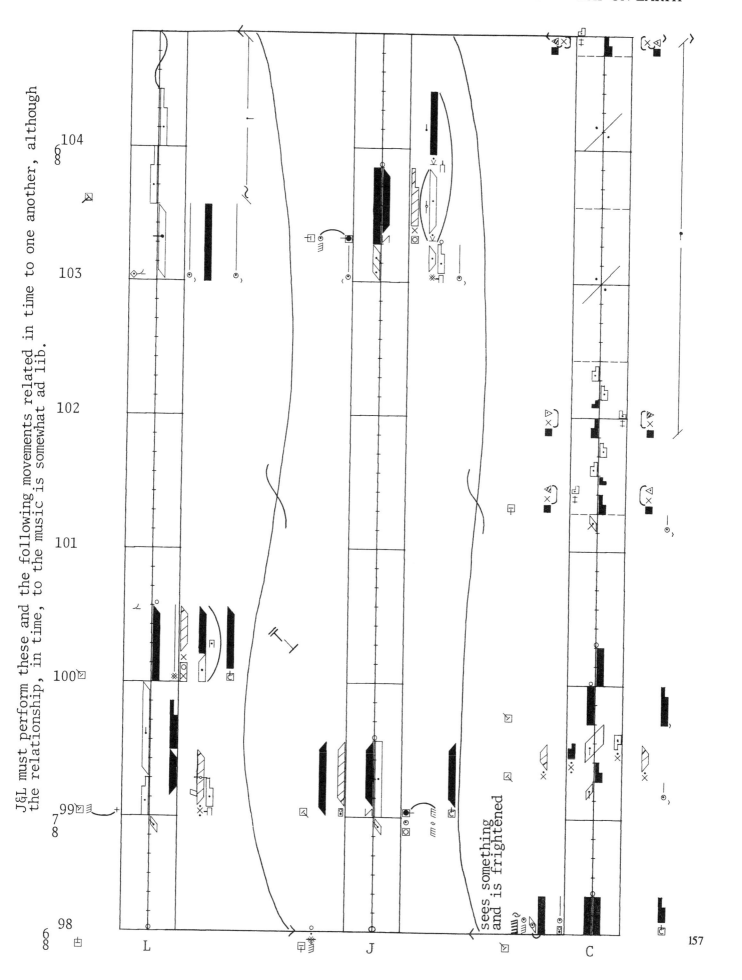

sees something and is frightened

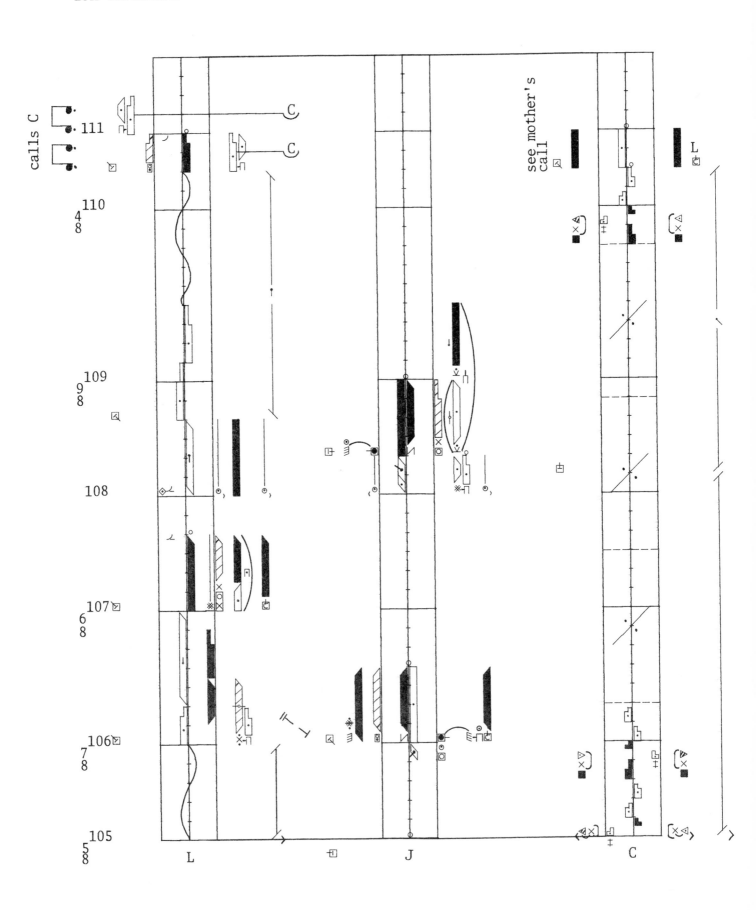

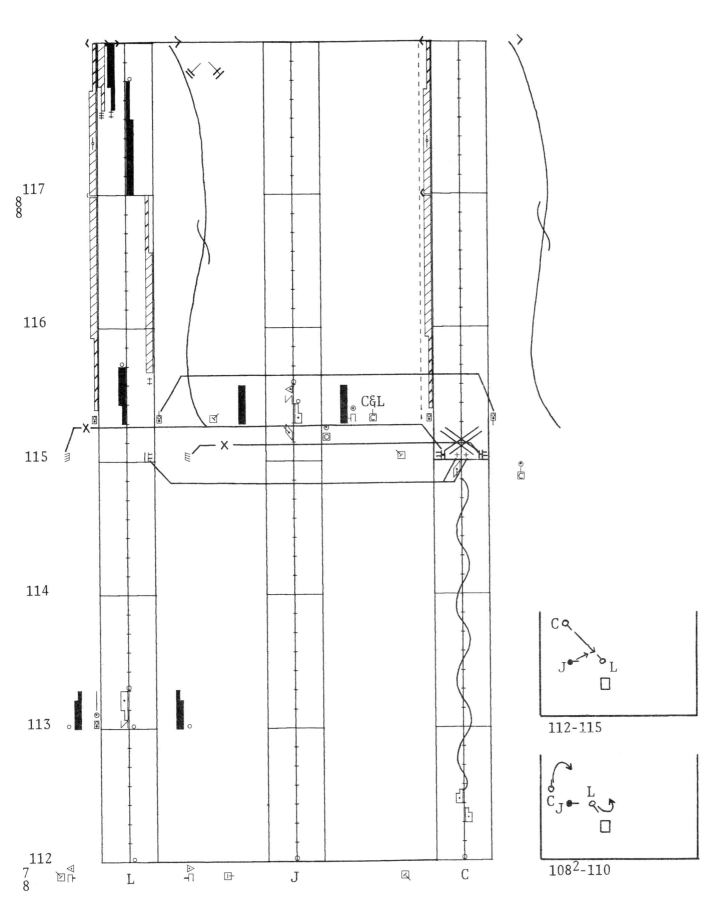

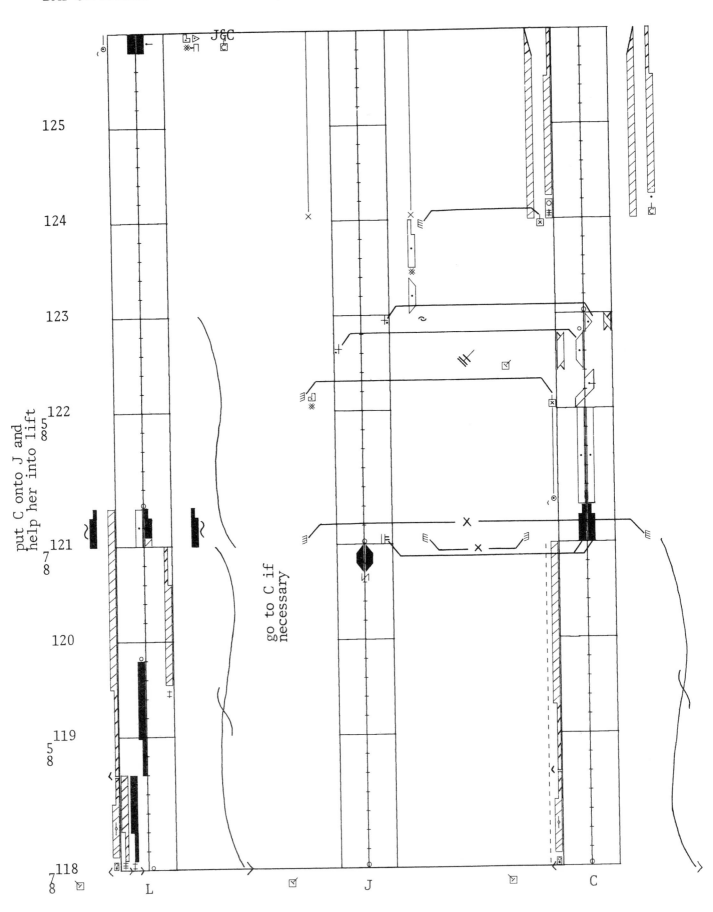

put C onto J and
help her into lift

go to C if
necessary

L   J   C

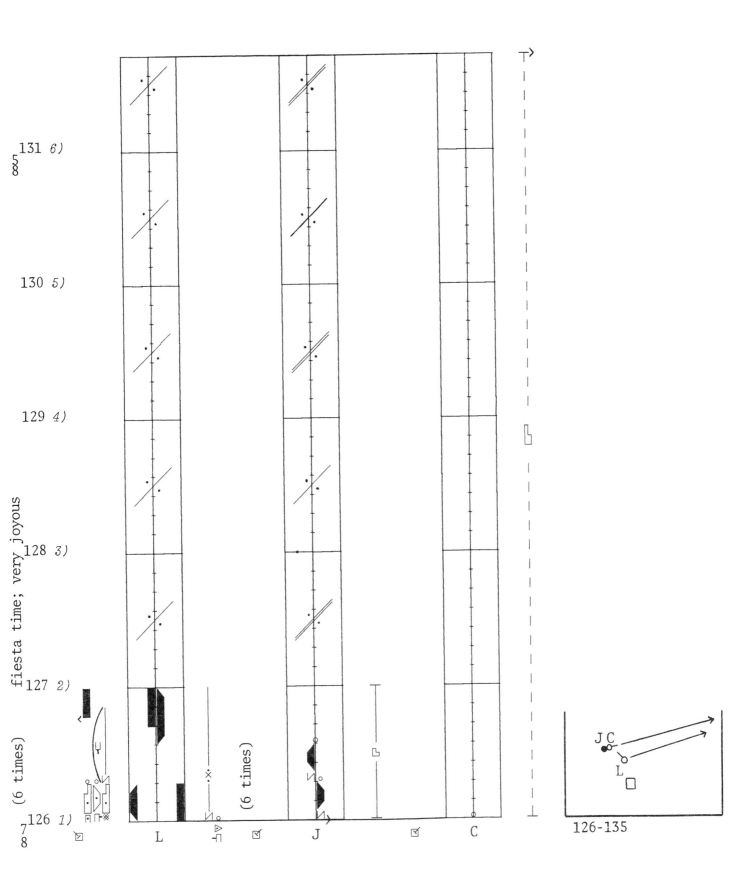

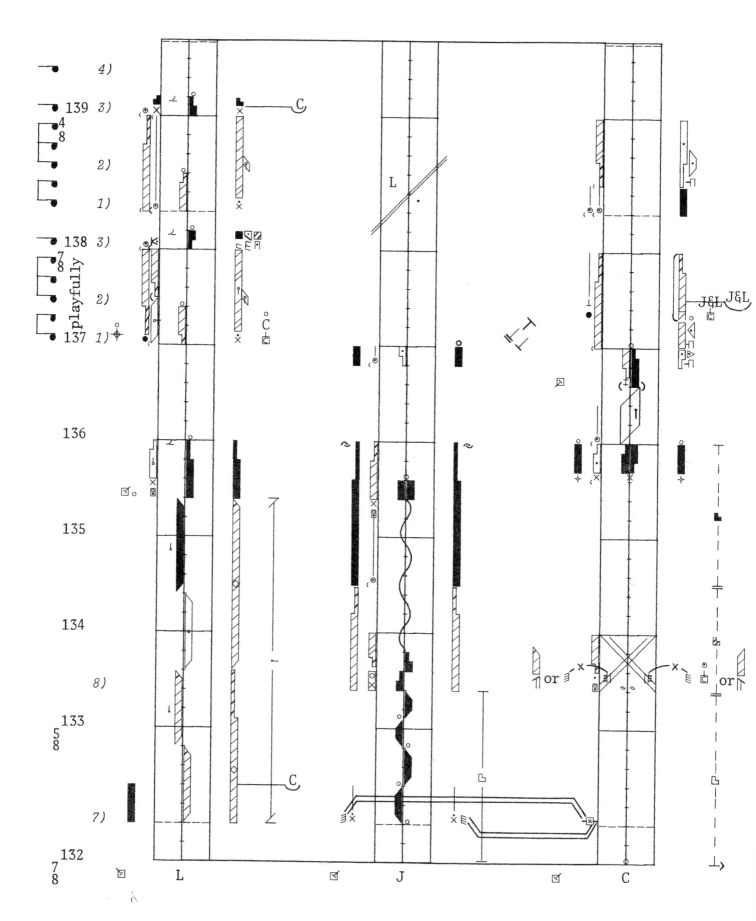

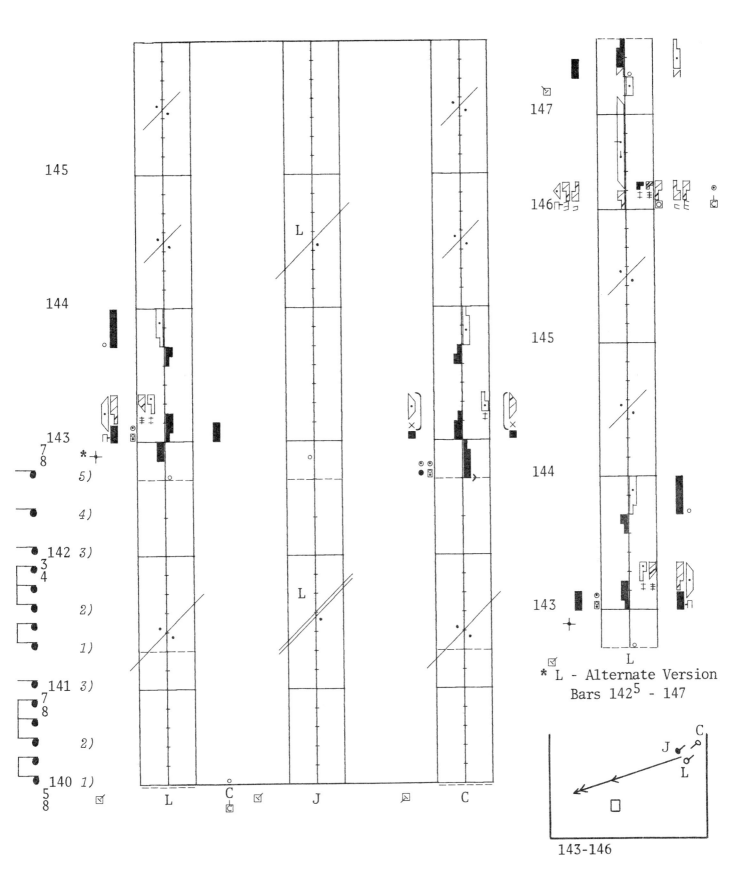

* L - Alternate Version
Bars 142^5 - 147

143-146

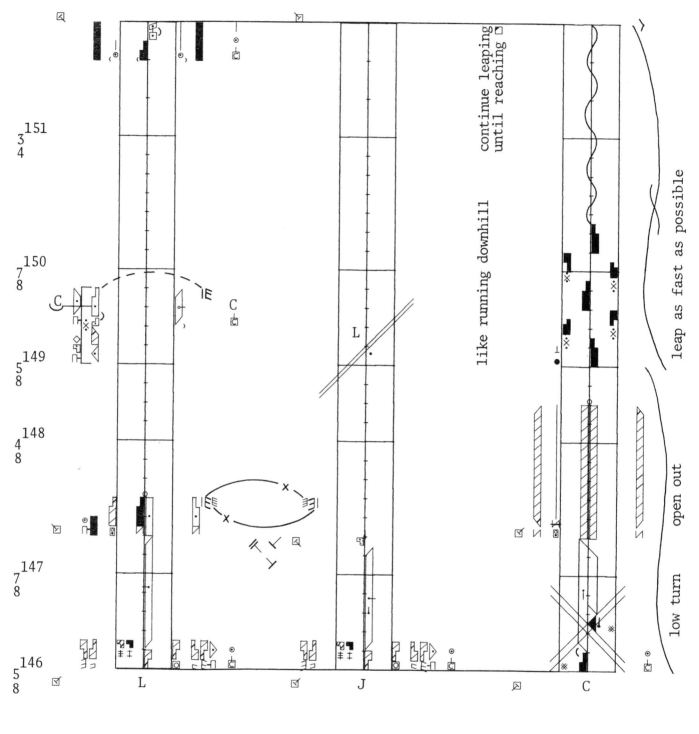

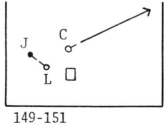

149-151

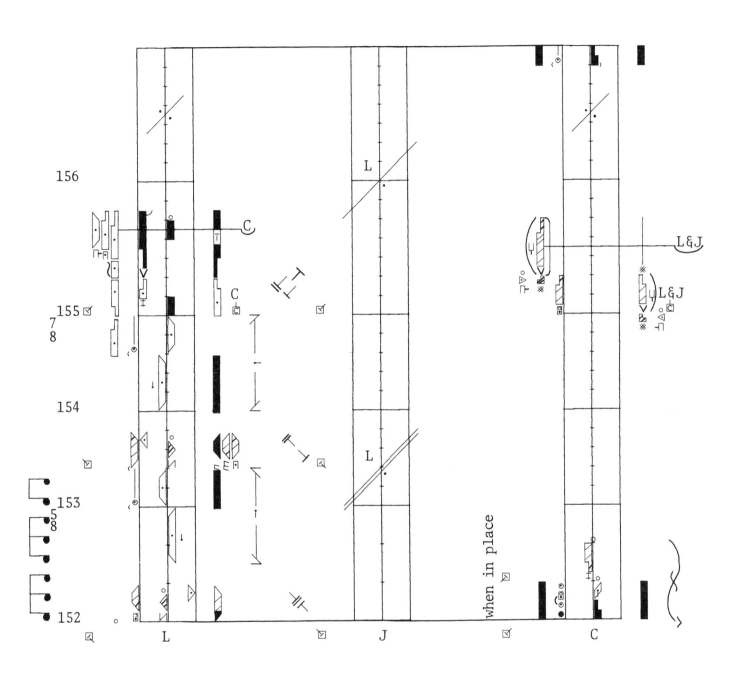

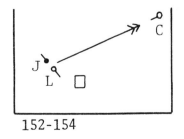

152-154

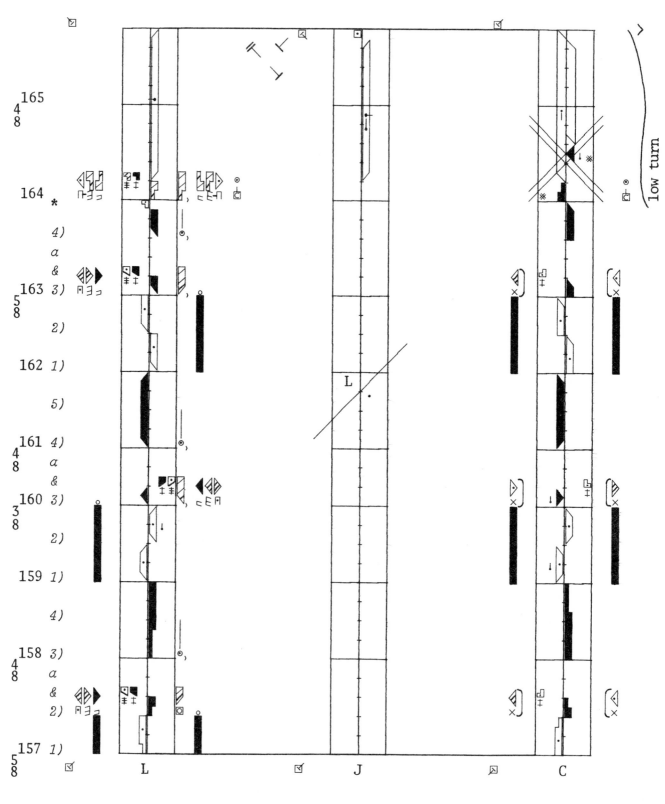

low turn

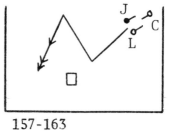

157-163

* For Alternate Version - L & J
   Bars 163^4 - 165 see Glossary.

Mother must leave for a while.
A moment of parting.

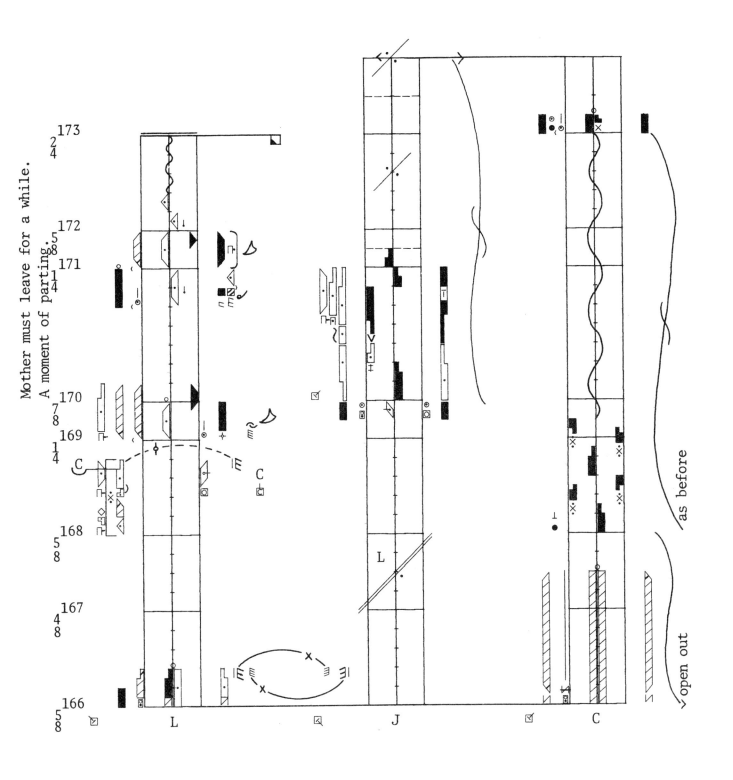

as before

open out

L   J   C

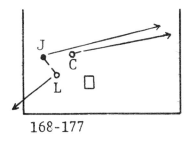

168-177

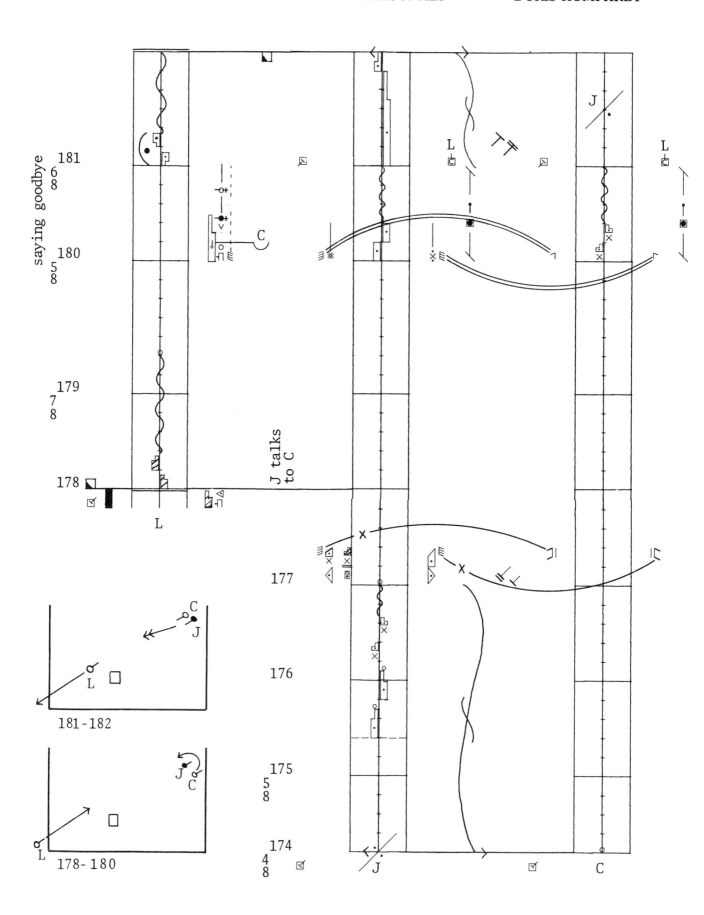

saying goodbye

181
6
8

180
5
8

179
7
8

178

J talks
to C

L

C

177

176

175
5
8

174
4
8

J   C

C
J

L   □

181-182

J
C

□

L
178-180

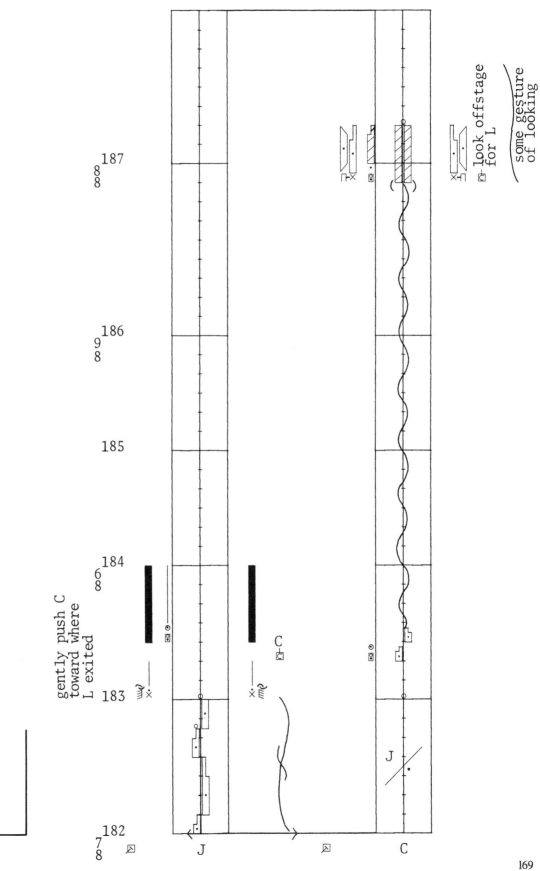

look offstage
for L

some gesture
of looking

187
8
8

186
9
8

185

184
6
8

gently push C
toward where
L exited

C

183

J

182
7
8

183-186

J

C

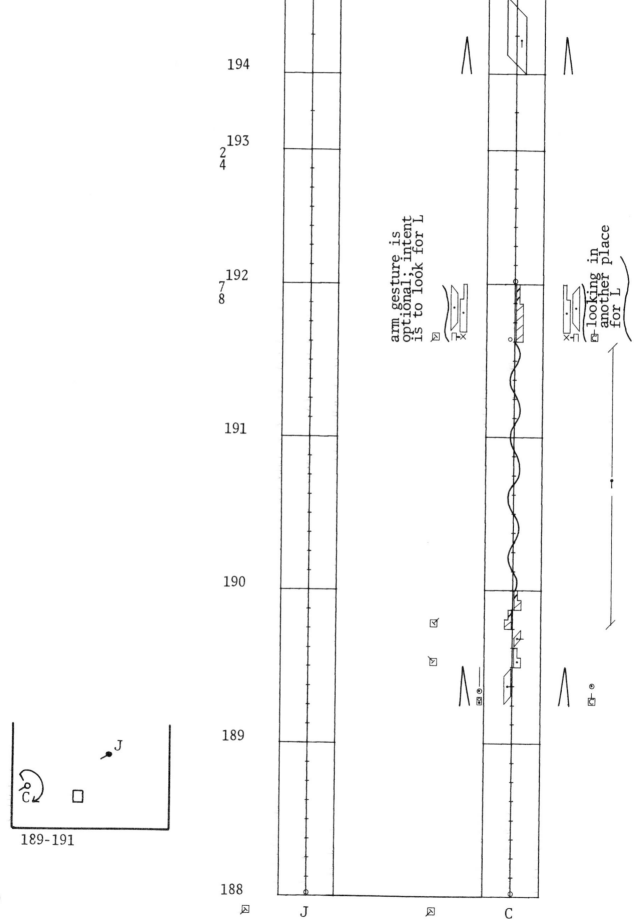

189-191

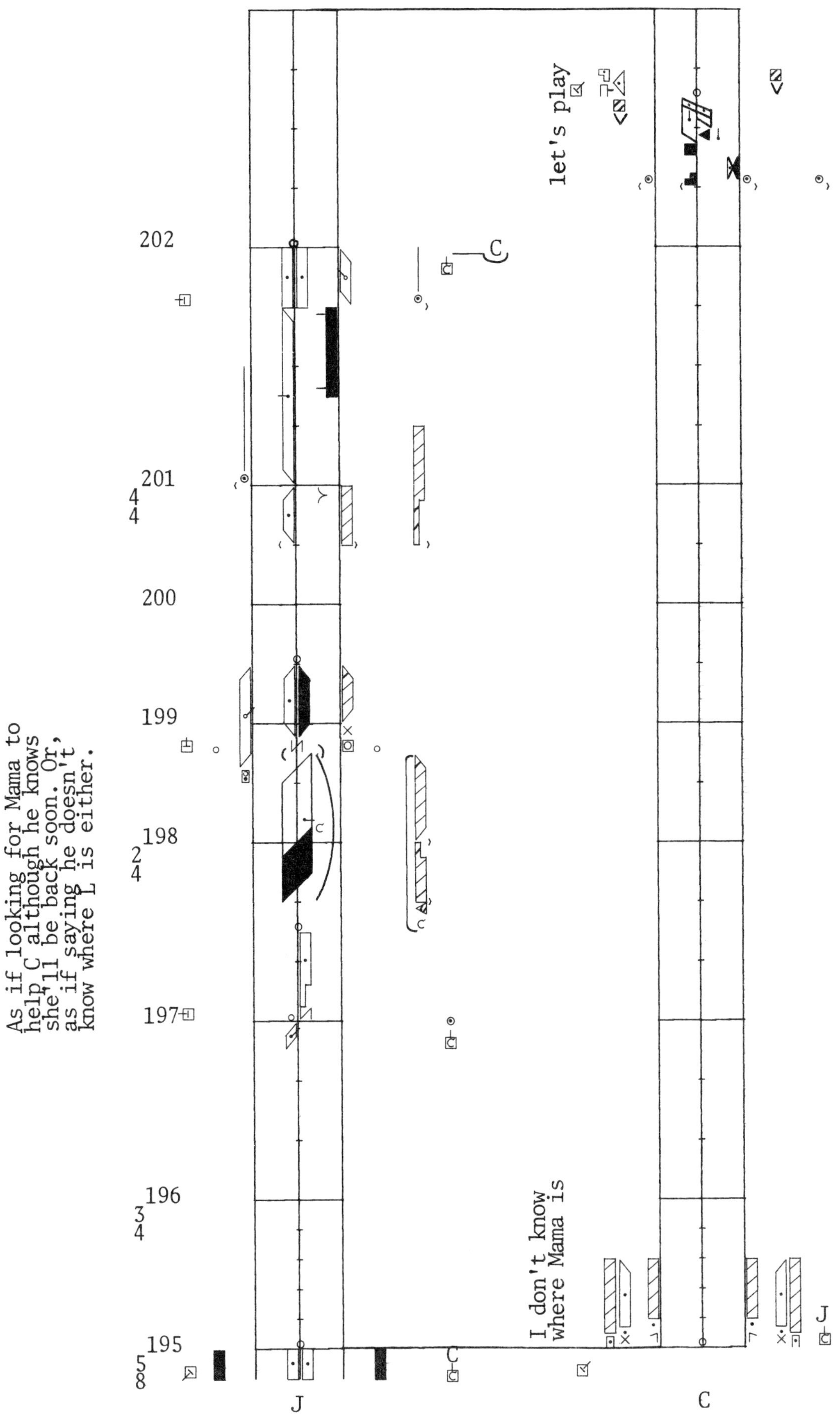

let's play

C

202

201

200

199

198

197

196

195

As if looking for Mama to
help C although he knows
she'll be back soon. Or,
as if saying he doesn't
know where L is either.

I don't know
where Mama is

J

C

J

C

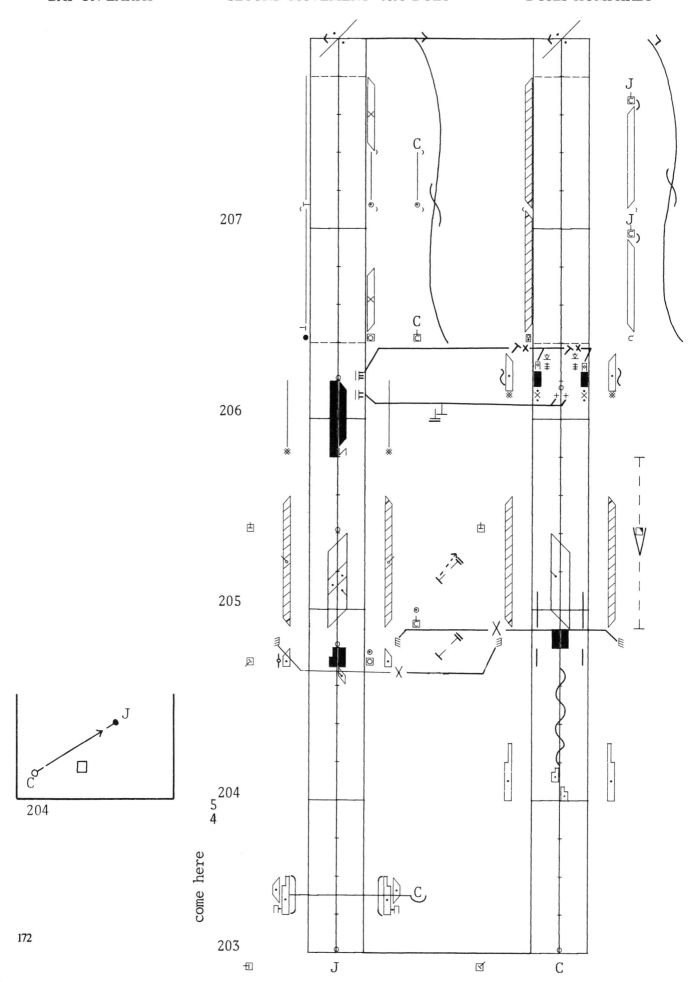

come here

207

206

205

204
5
4

203

204

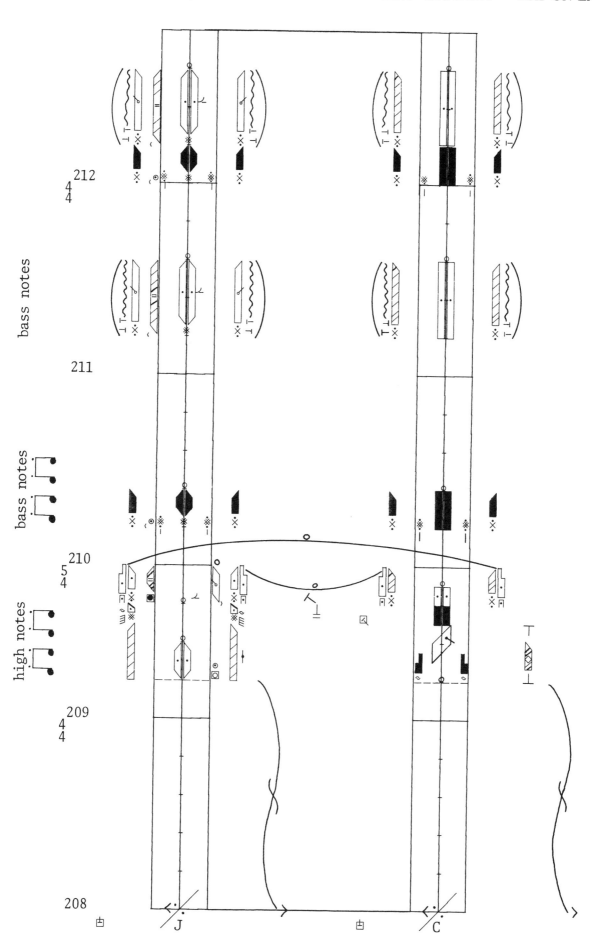

bass notes

bass notes

high notes

212

4
4

211

210

5
4

209

4
4

208

J

C

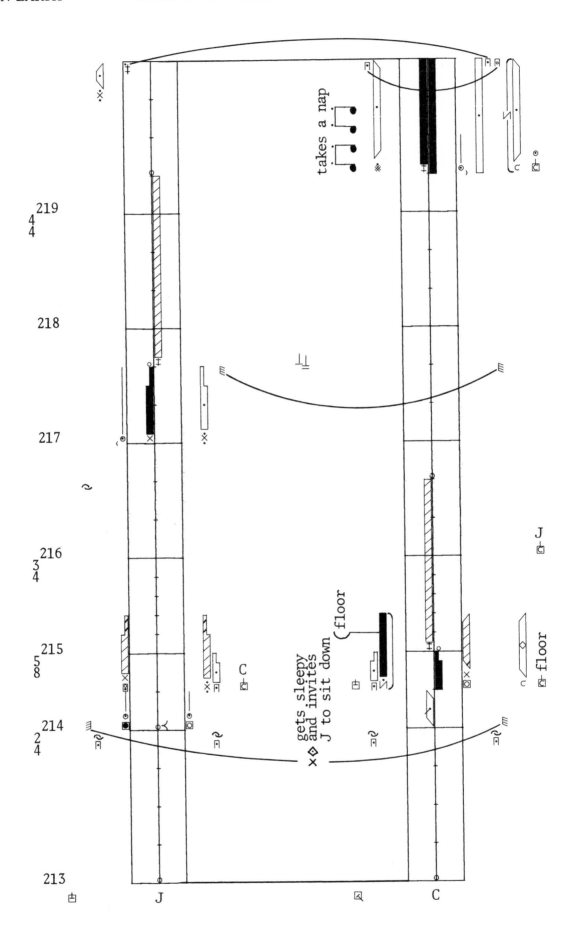

takes a nap

floor

gets sleepy
and invites
J to sit down

C

floor

J

219
4
4

218

217

216
3
4

215
5
8

214
2
4

213

J

C

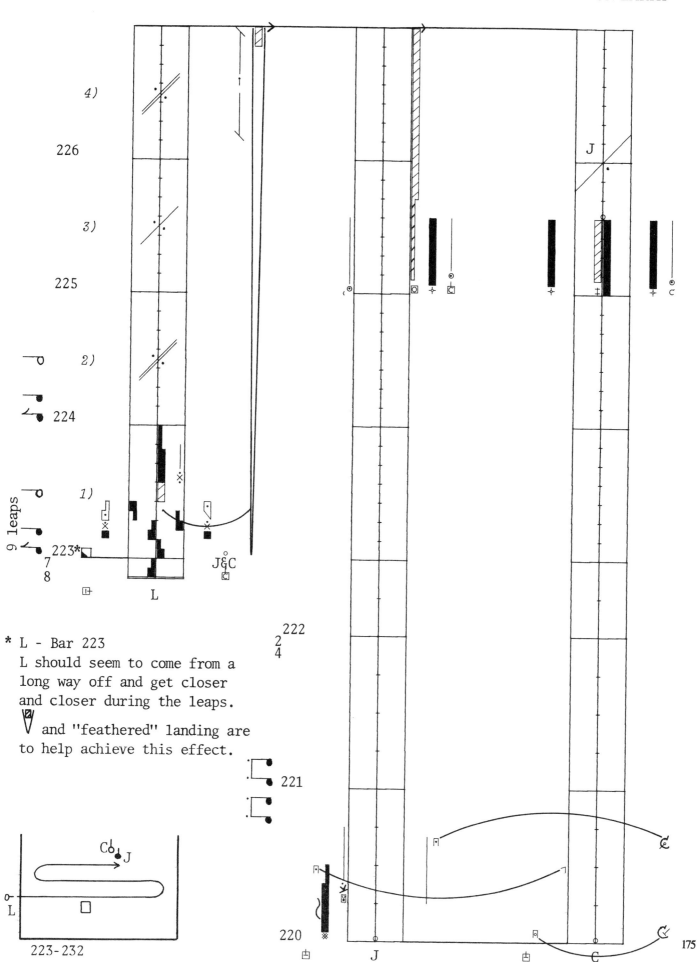

4)

226

3)

225

2)

224

9 leaps

1)

7
8

223*

J&C

L

* L - Bar 223
  L should seem to come from a
  long way off and get closer
  and closer during the leaps.

  and "feathered" landing are
  to help achieve this effect.

221

C♭
J

L

223-232

222
2
4

220

J

C

175

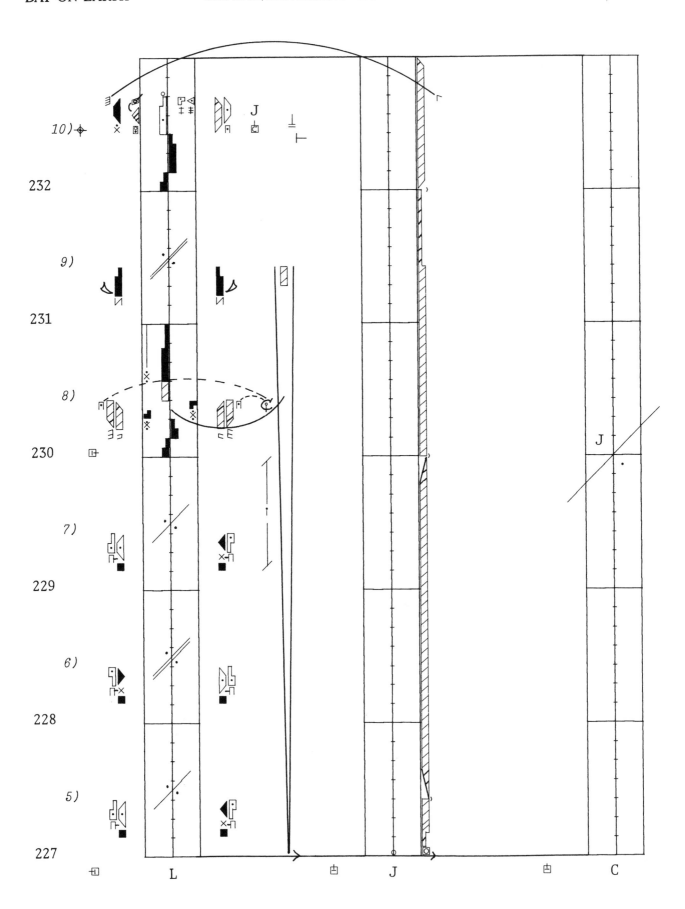

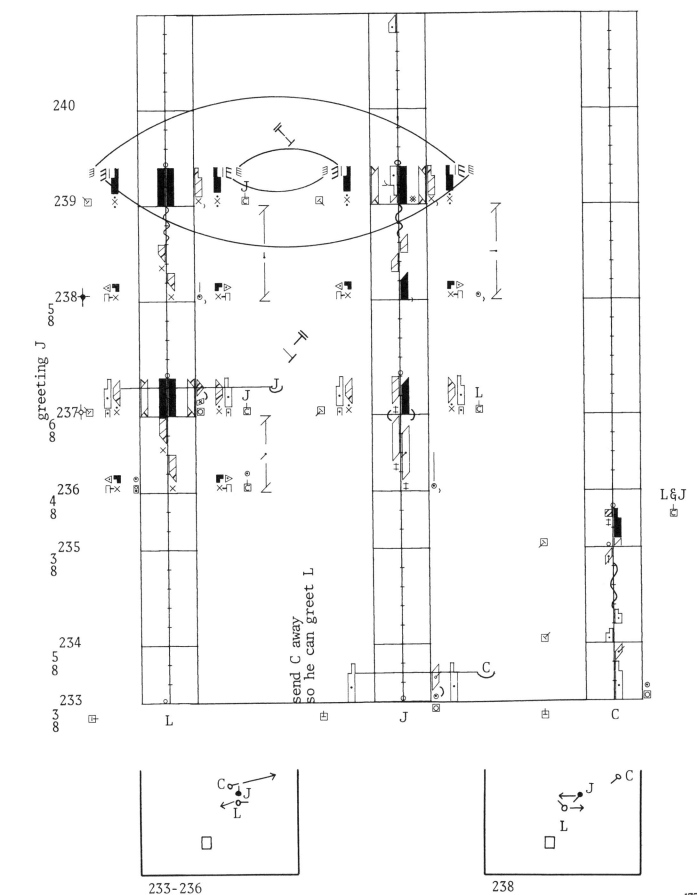

233-236   238

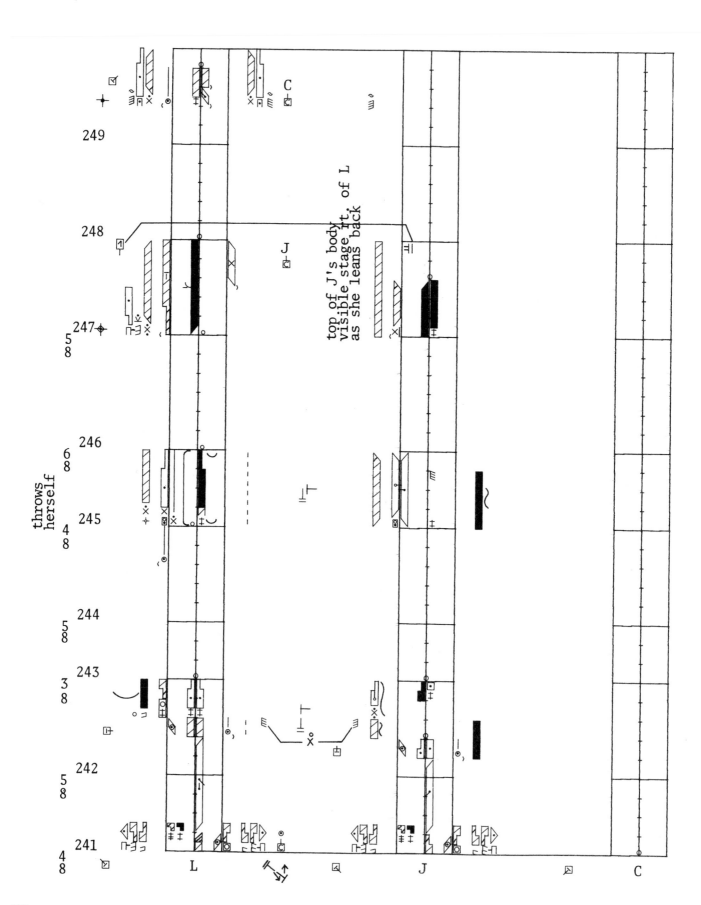

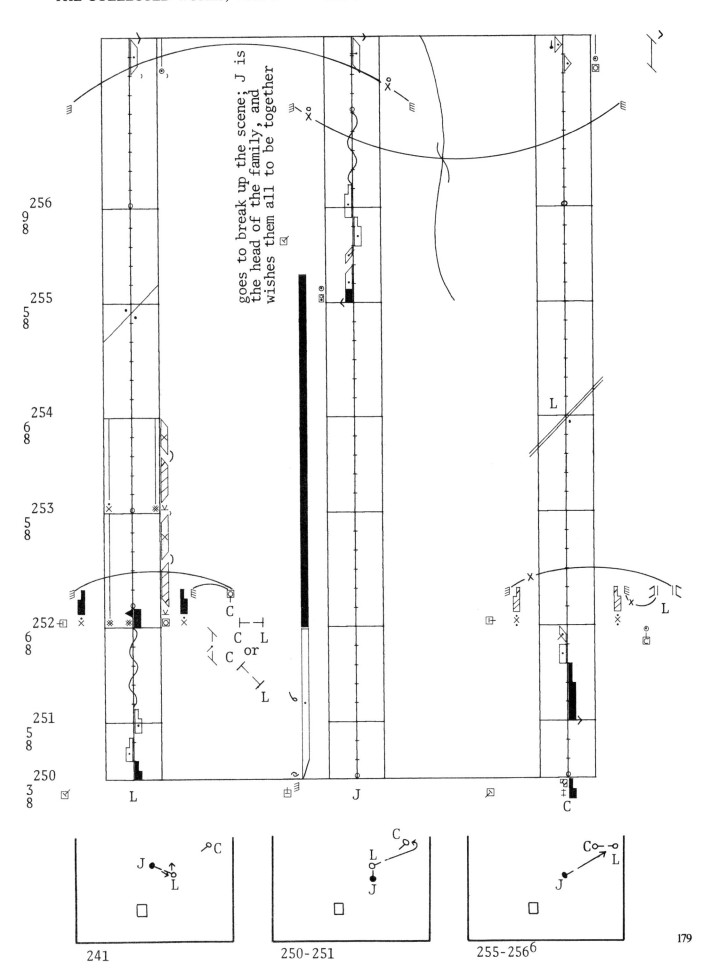

goes to break up the scene; J is
the head of the family, and
wishes them all to be together

C
C   L
C   or
    L

L   J   C

241   250-251   255-256

179

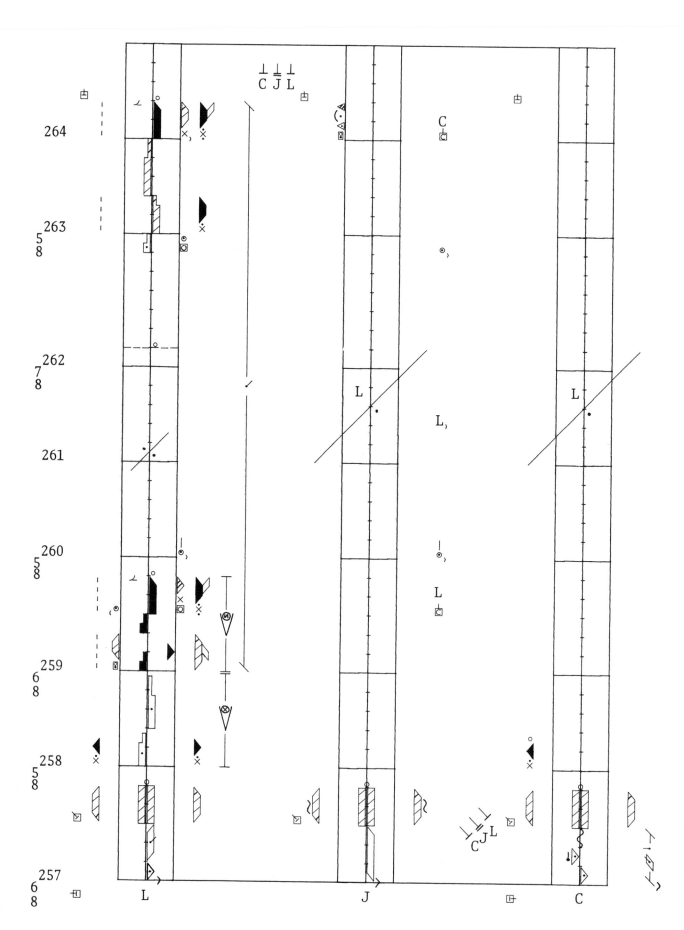

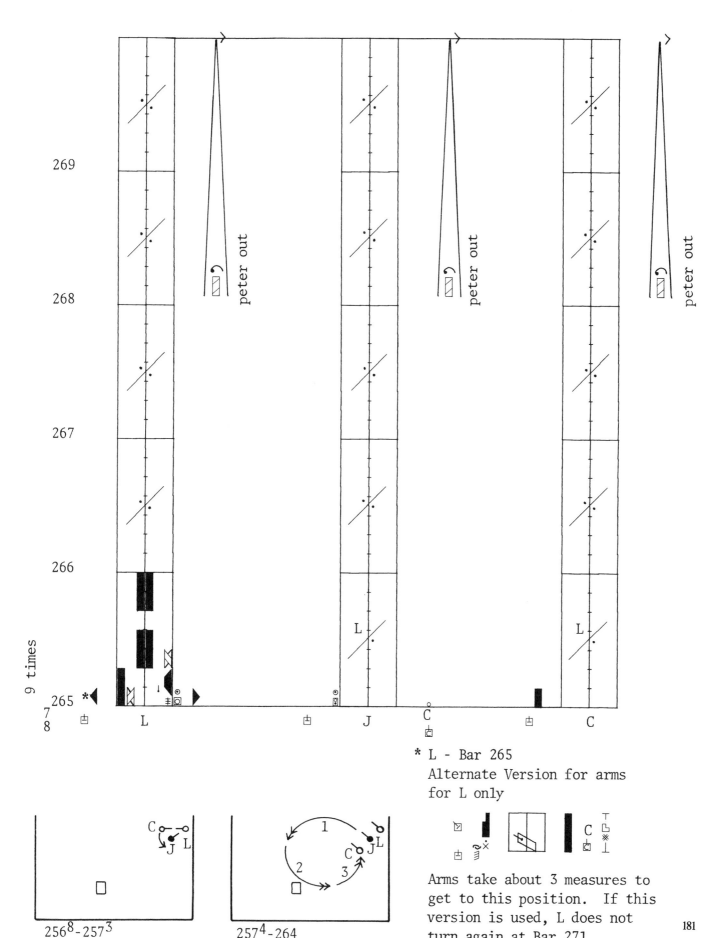

9 times

269

268

267

266

265

7
8

peter out

peter out

peter out

L

L

L

J

C

C

* L - Bar 265
Alternate Version for arms
for L only

Arms take about 3 measures to
get to this position. If this
version is used, L does not
turn again at Bar 271.

C L
J

C J L
1
2 3

256⁸-257³

257⁴-264

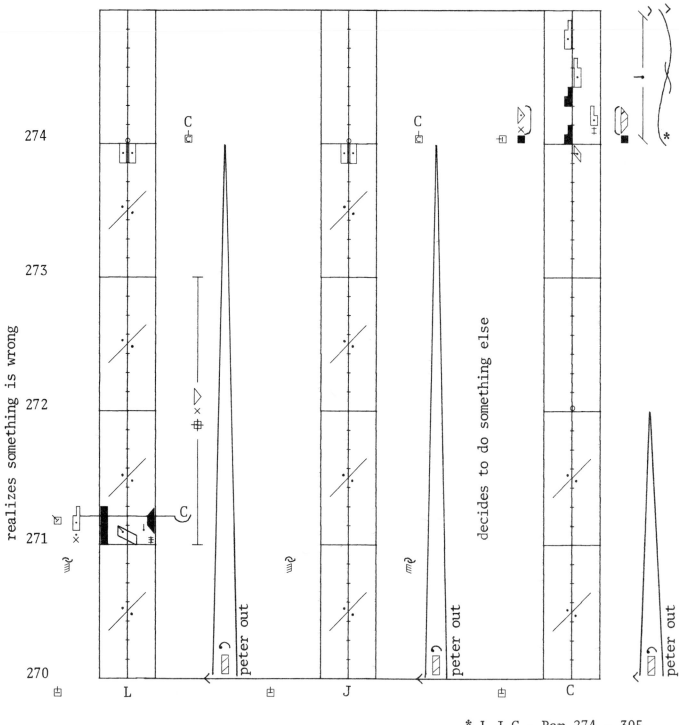

realizes something is wrong

decides to do something else

274

273

272

271

270

L   J   C

peter out   peter out   peter out

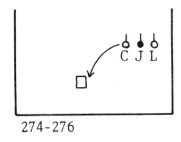

C J L

274-276

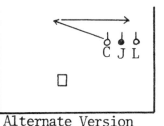

C J L

Alternate Version
in film

Note: On early film C
does a different path.
The path is open to
interpretation.

* L,J,C - Bar 274 - 305
The timing is ad lib and is
performed on sight cues.
Movement which is written
simultaneously happens at
the same time for all 3
dancers but not necessarily
in the exact music bar in
which it is notated.

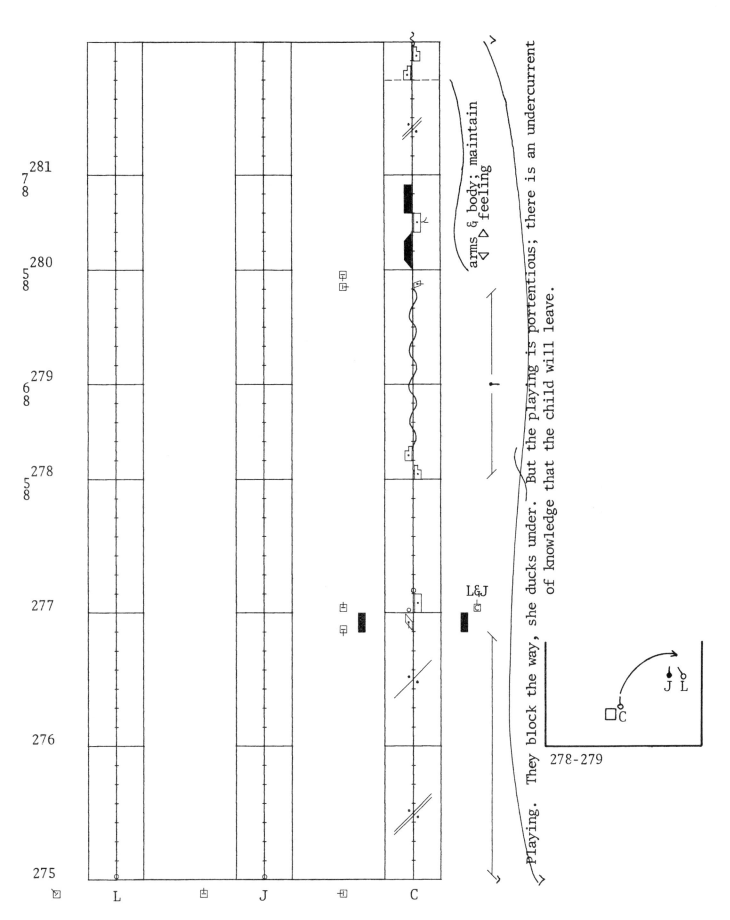

arms & body; maintain feeling

Playing. They block the way, she ducks under. But the playing is portentious; there is an undercurrent of knowledge that the child will leave.

L&J

278-279

J L

C

L   J   C

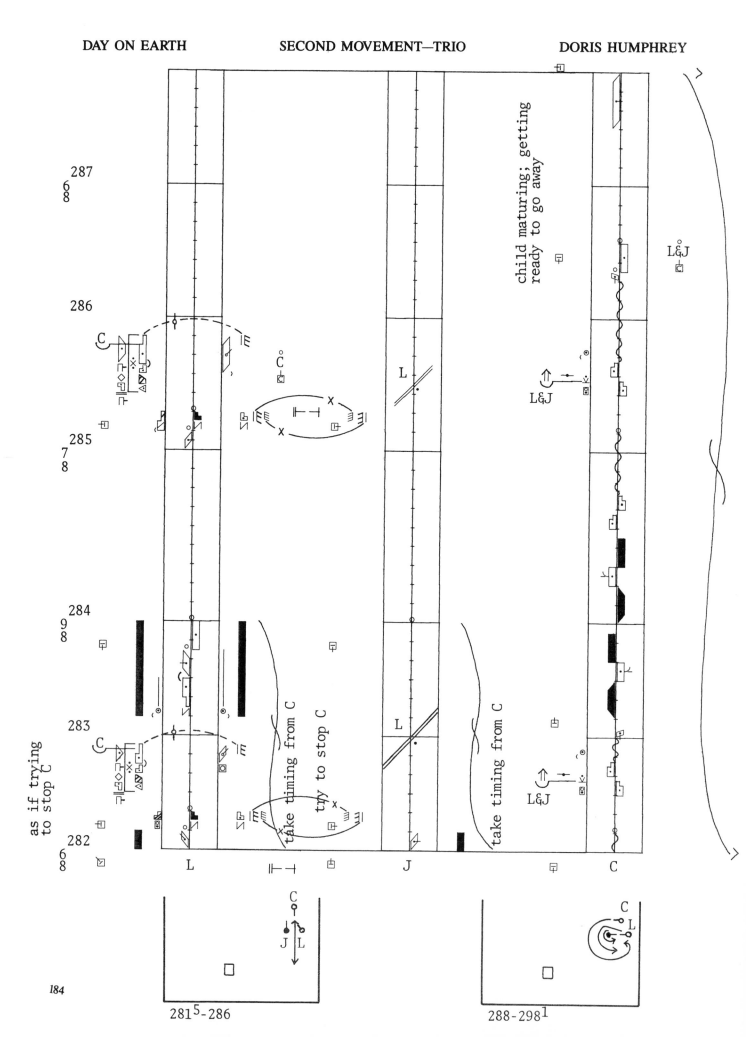

child maturing; getting
ready to go away

L&J

L&J

L&J

take timing from C

try to stop C

take timing from C

as if trying
to stop C

287
6
8

286

285
7
8

284
9
8

283

282
6
8

184

L&J

L

L

C

C

L

J

C

281⁵-286

288-298¹

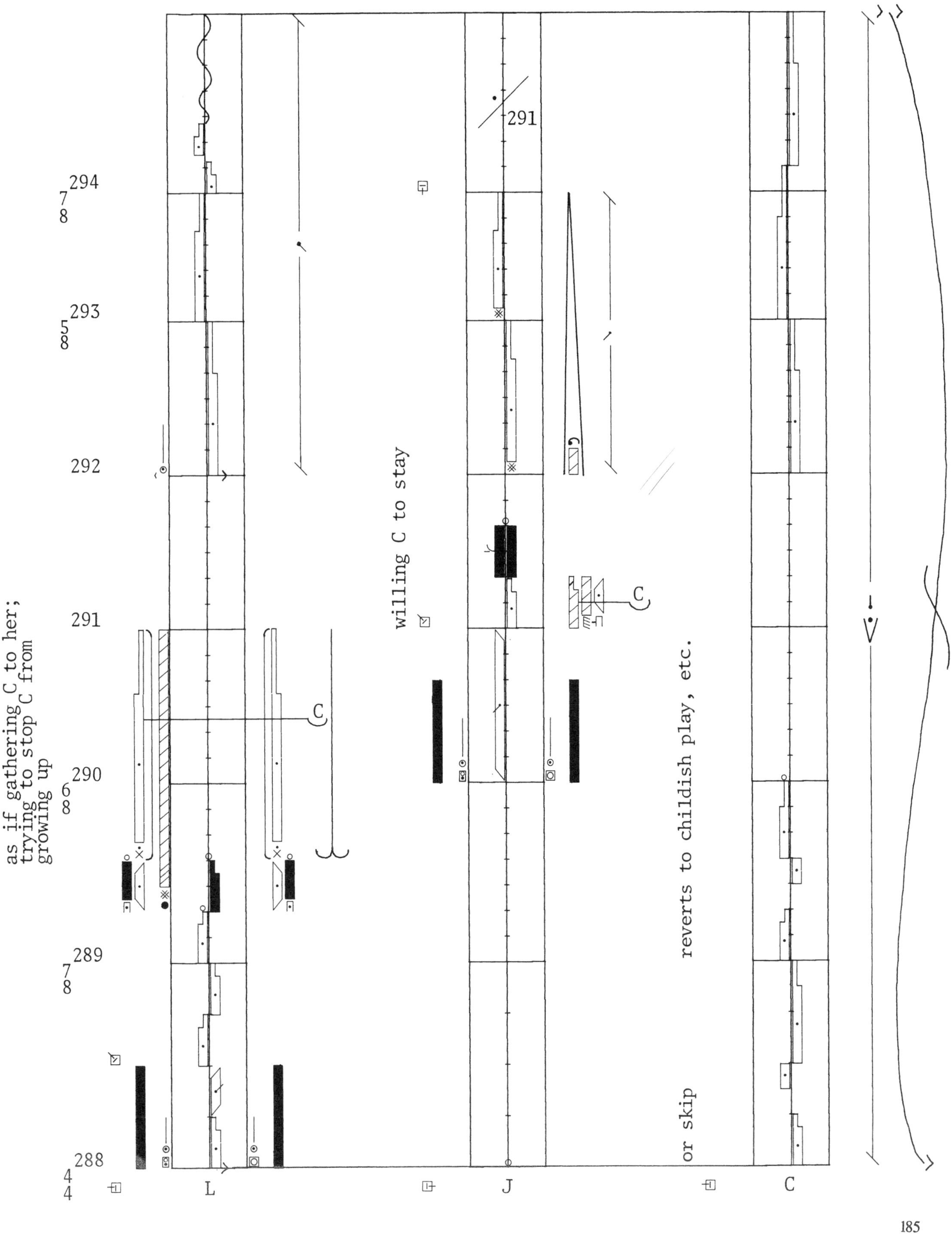

288
289
290
291
292
293
294
4
4
7
8
6
8
5
8
7
8
as if gathering C to her; trying to stop C from growing up
C
willing C to stay
291
C
reverts to childish play, etc.
or skip
L
J
C

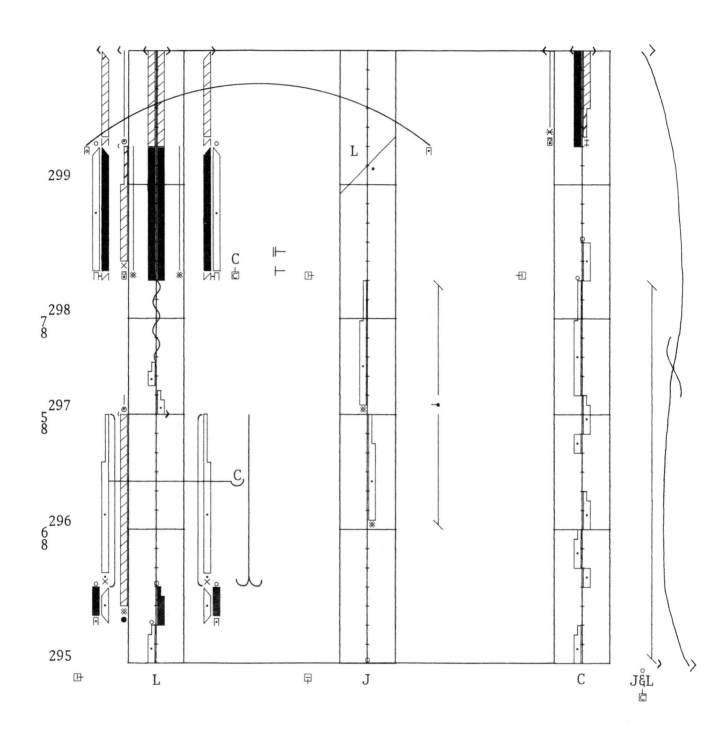

299

298
7
8

297
5
8

296
6
8

295

L   J   C   J&L

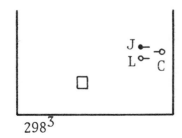

298³

* L&J - Bar 306 - Transition
  As if retreating. As C grows up,
  parents seem to get smaller.
  Walk is weighty, sorrowful, and
  one long descent to knees.
  (See page 76.)
  Letitia Ide remembers this as
  being further downstage.

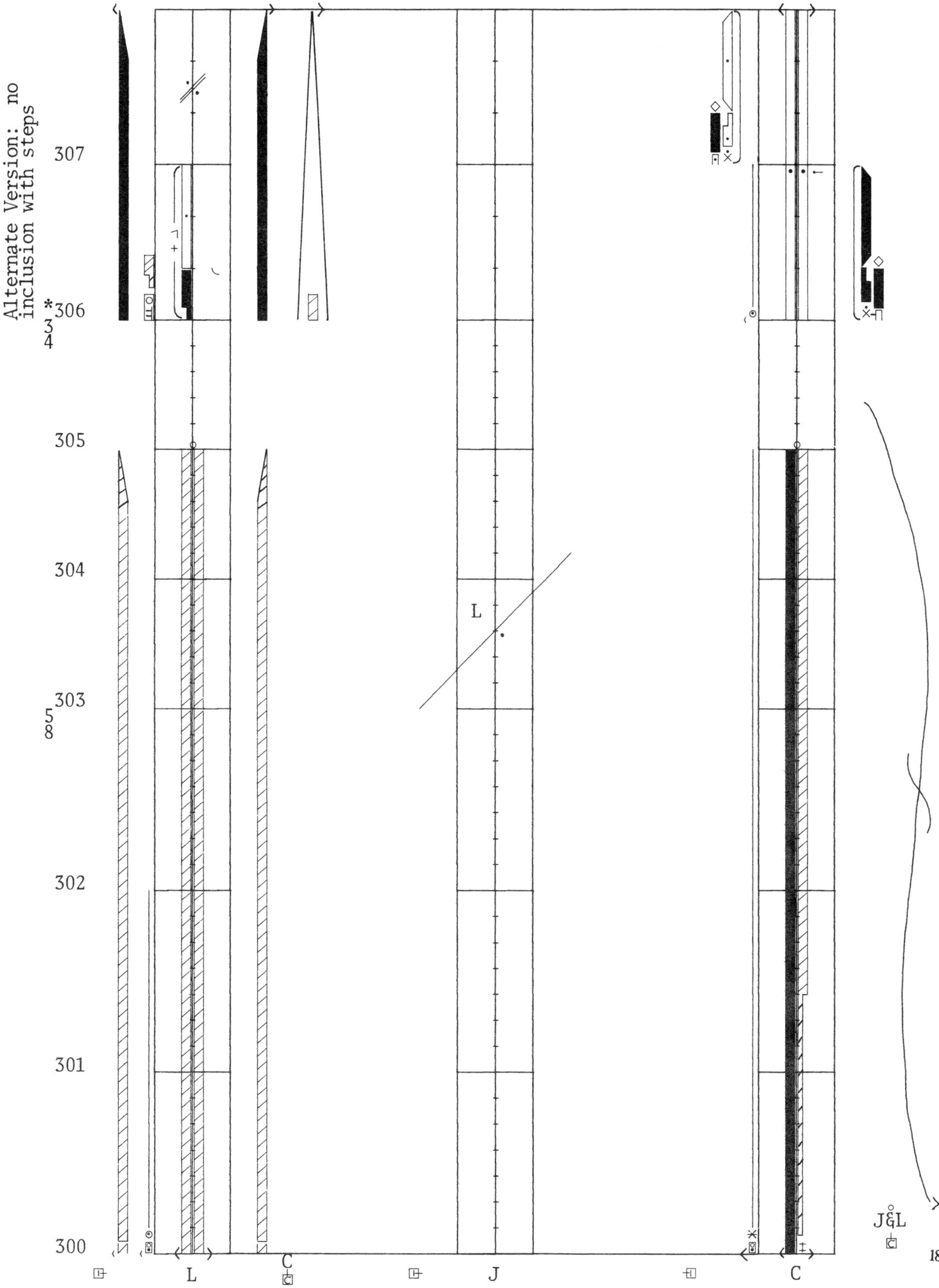
Alternate Version: no inclusion with steps
307
*306
3
4
305
304
L
303
5
8
302
301
300
L
C
J
C
J&L

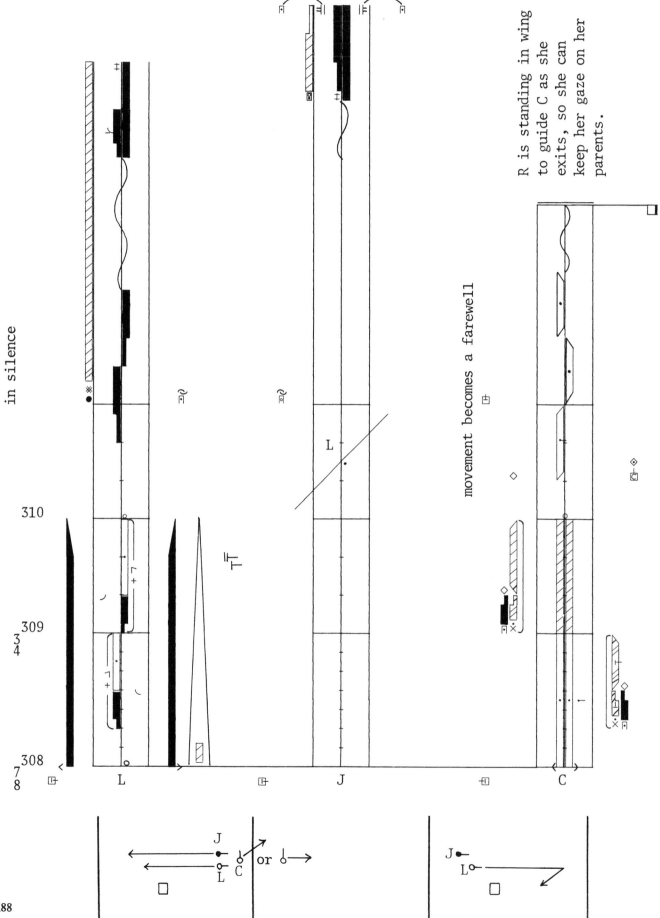

in silence

R is standing in wing to guide C as she exits, so she can keep her gaze on her parents.

movement becomes a farewell

310

309

308

L J C

306-Silence 3^2-7

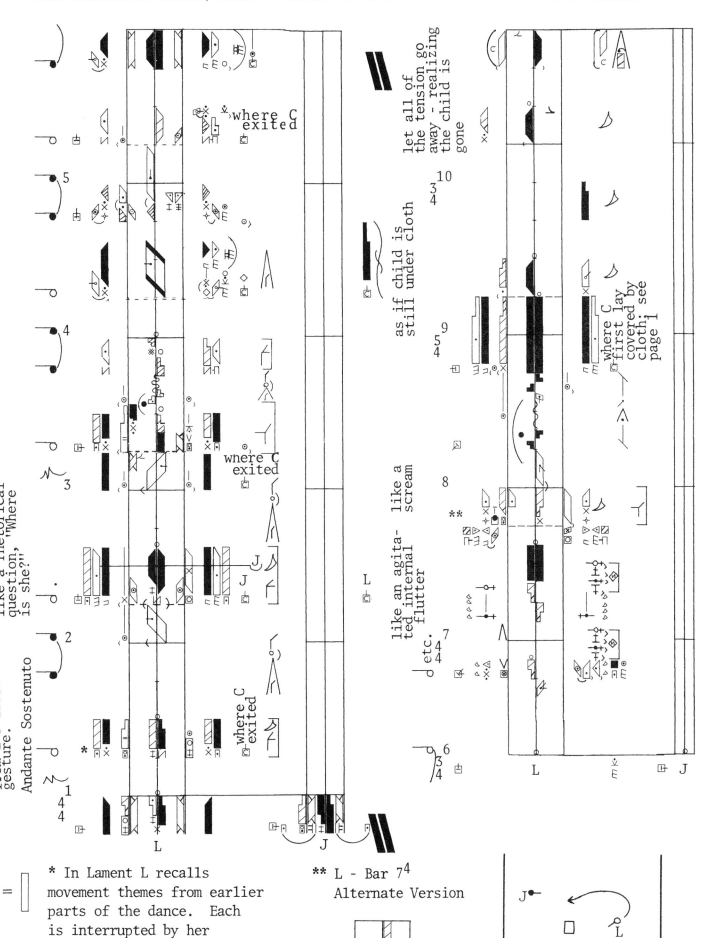

like a rhetorical question, "Where is she?"

Pianist takes cue from L's first gesture.

Andante Sostenuto

where C exited

where C exited

where C exited

J

let all of the tension go away - realizing the child is gone

as if child is still under cloth

like a scream

like an agitated internal flutter

etc.

where C first lay covered by cloth; see page 1

L

* In Lament L recalls movement themes from earlier parts of the dance. Each is interrupted by her realization that the child is no longer with her.

** L - Bar 7⁴ Alternate Version

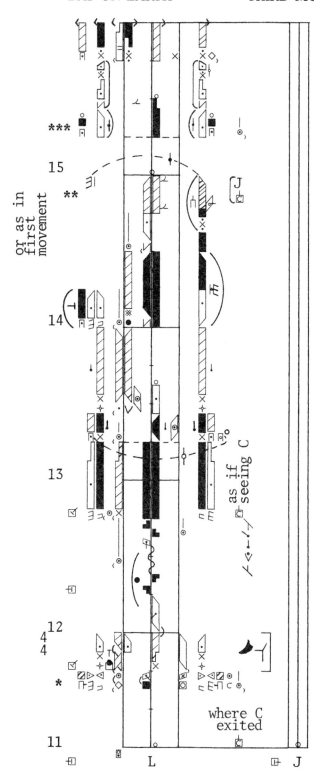

*** L - Bar 15²-16²
Alternate Version for
supports; arms and body
remain as written

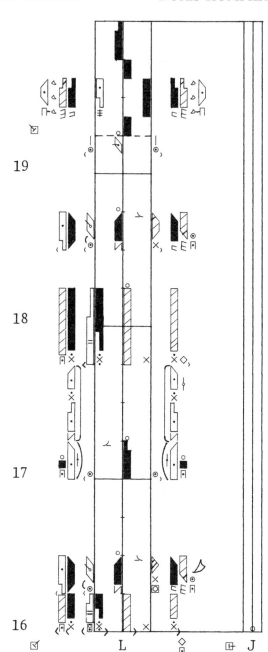

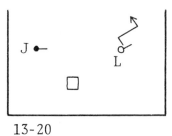

13-20

Or as in
first
movement

as if
seeing C

where C
exited

** L - Bar 14⁴
   is optional. This is one
    possible interpretation.

* L - Bar 11²⁻³
  Alternate Version

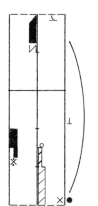

12

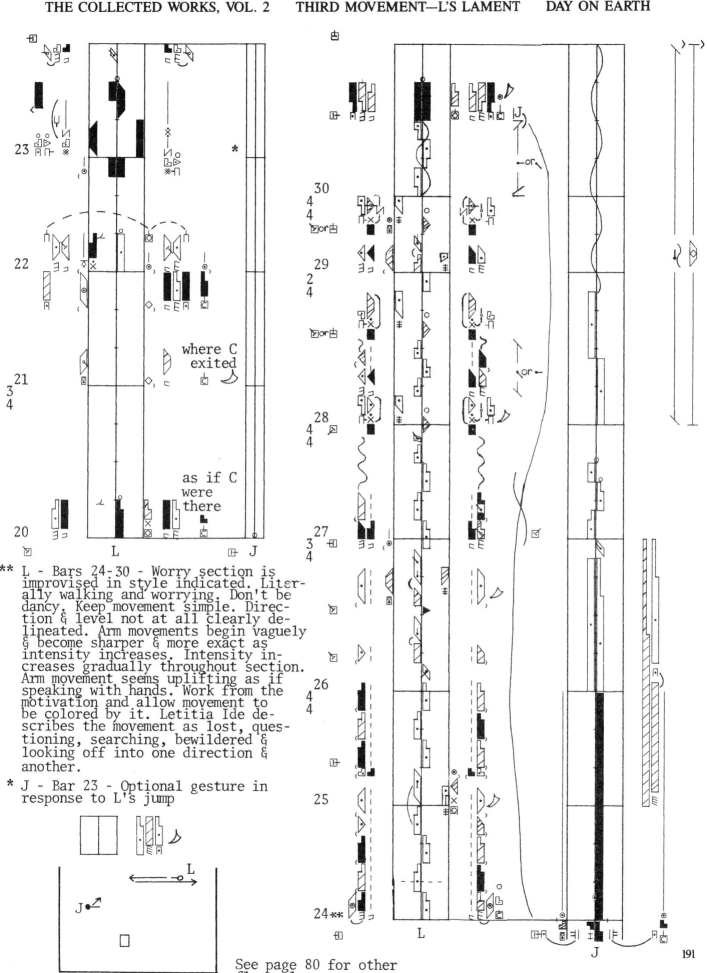

** L - Bars 24-30 - Worry section is improvised in style indicated. Literally walking and worrying. Don't be dancy. Keep movement simple. Direction & level not at all clearly delineated. Arm movements begin vaguely & become sharper & more exact as intensity increases. Intensity increases gradually throughout section. Arm movement seems uplifting as if speaking with hands. Work from the motivation and allow movement to be colored by it. Letitia Ide describes the movement as lost, questioning, searching, bewildered & looking off into one direction & another.

* J - Bar 23 - Optional gesture in response to L's jump

where C exited

as if C were there

See page 80 for other floor plan.

24-26

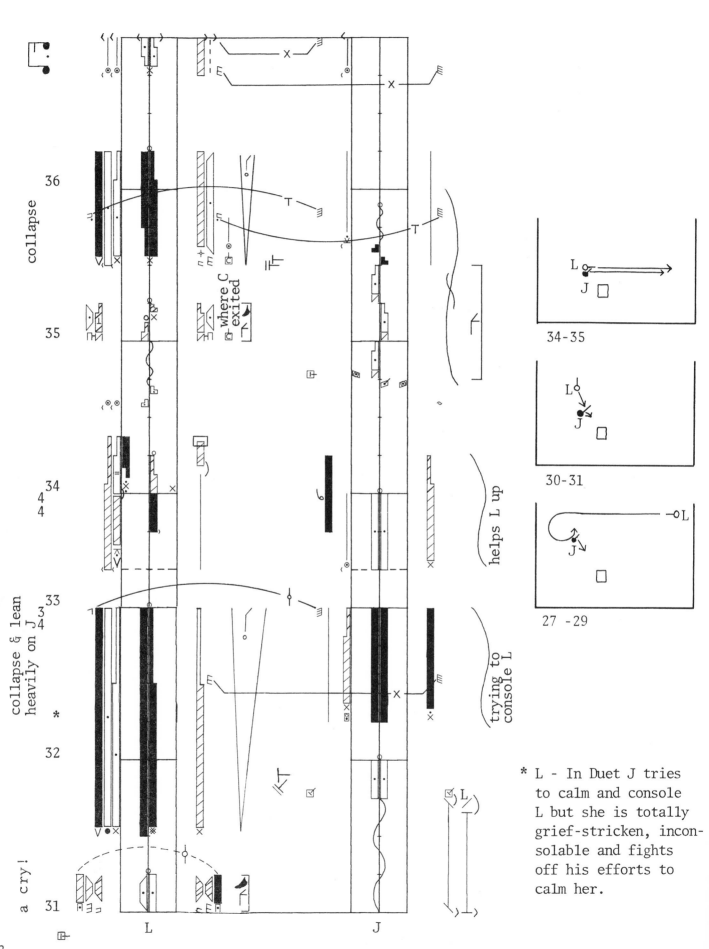

34-35

30-31

27 -29

* L - In Duet J tries
to calm and console
L but she is totally
grief-stricken, incon-
solable and fights
off his efforts to
calm her.

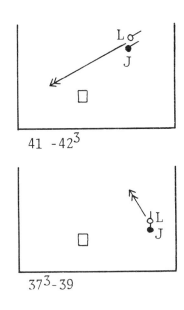

41 -42³

37³-39

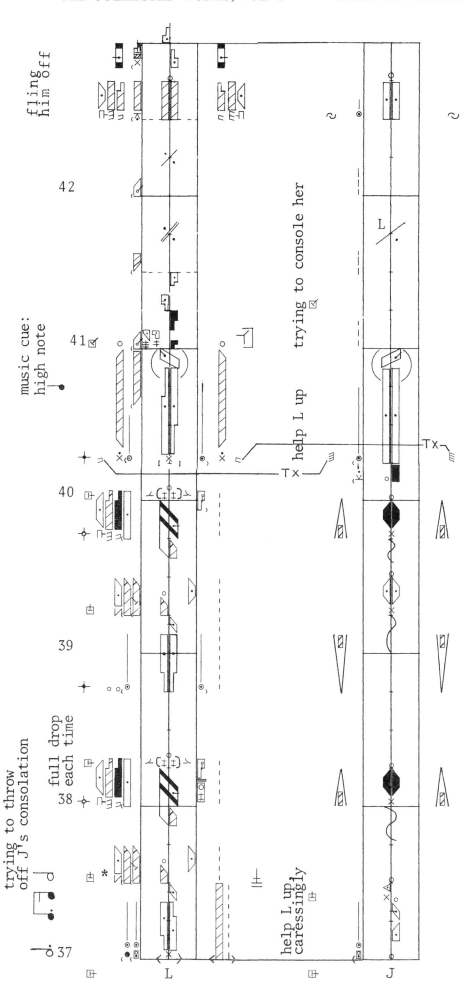

fling
him off

42

music cue:
high note

41

trying to console her

help L up

40

Tx

39

full drop
each time

trying to throw
off J's consolation

38

help L up
caressingly

37

L

J

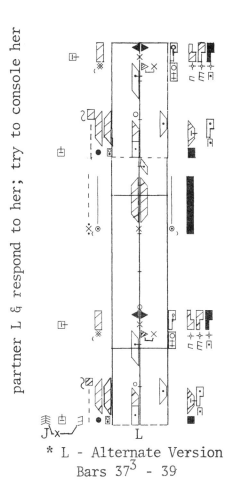

partner L & respond to her; try to console her

L

* L - Alternate Version
Bars 37³ - 39

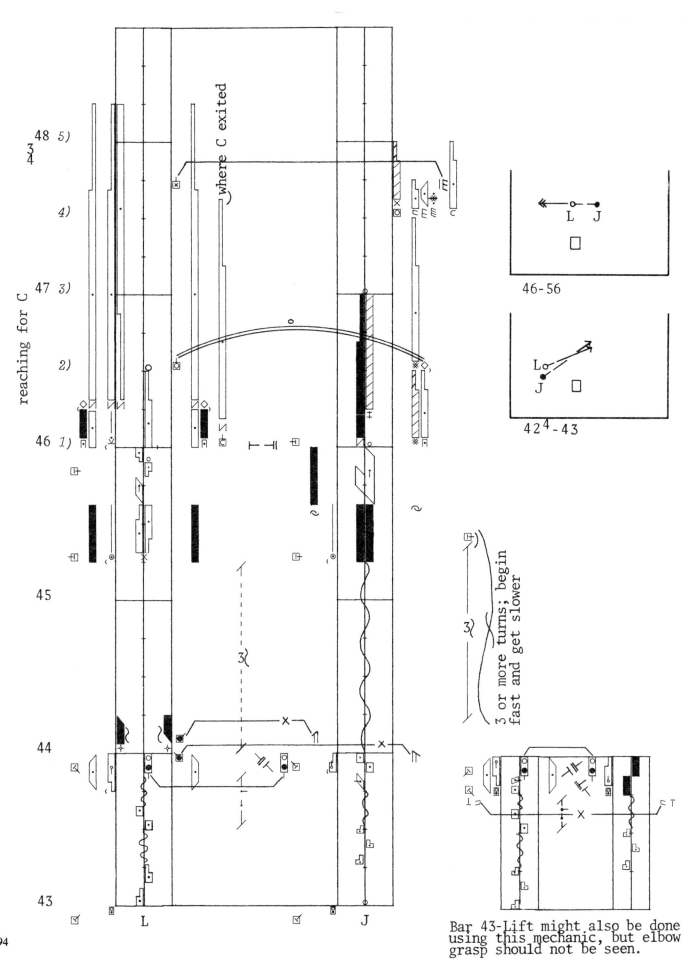

reaching for C

where C exited

48 5)
3
4

4)

47 3)

2)

46 1)

45

44

43

L   J

46-56

42⁴-43

3 or more turns; begin
fast and get slower

3{

Bar 43-Lift might also be done
using this mechanic, but elbow
grasp should not be seen.

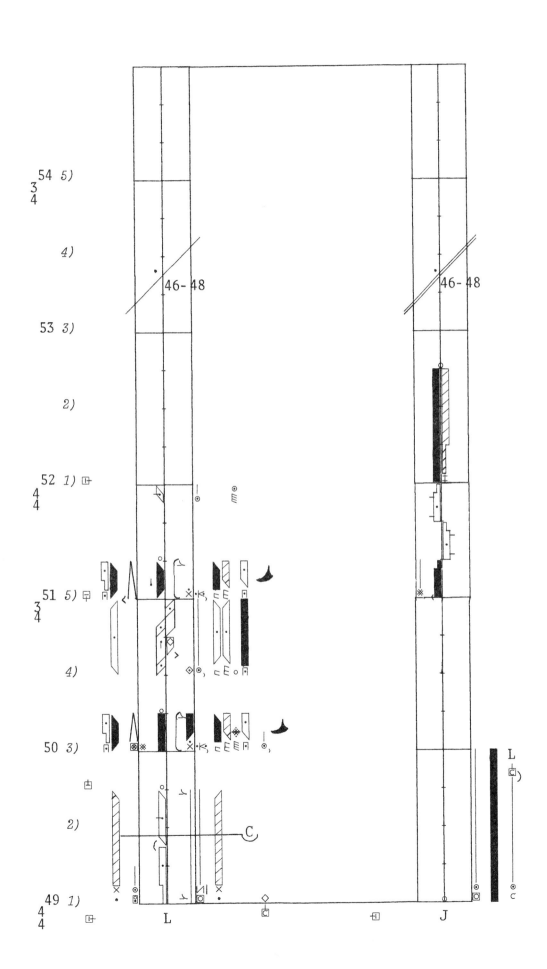

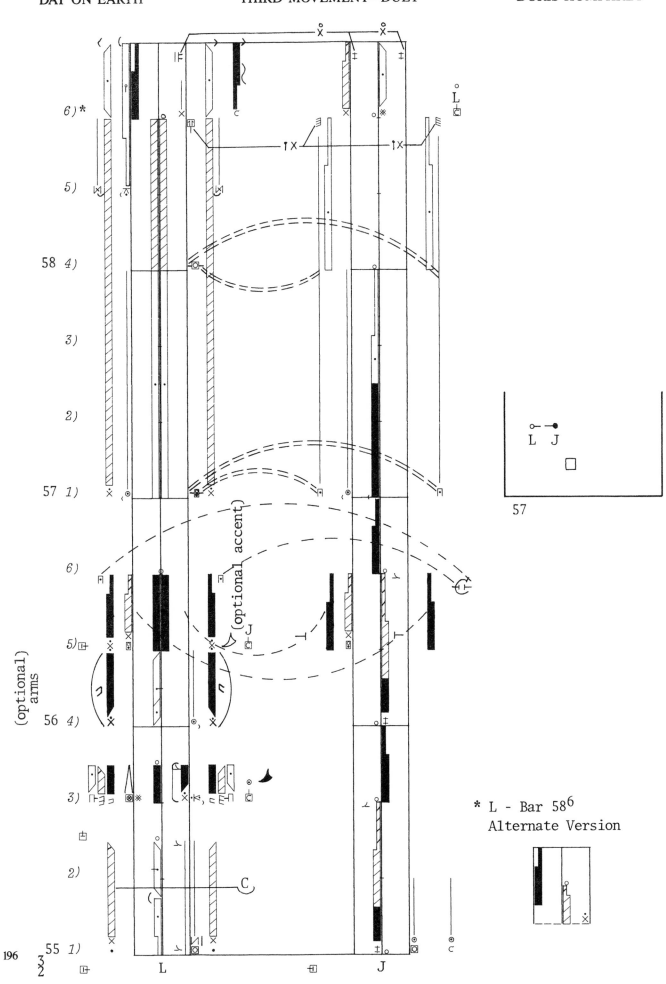

(optional accent)

(optional) arms

L   J

57

* L - Bar 58⁶
Alternate Version

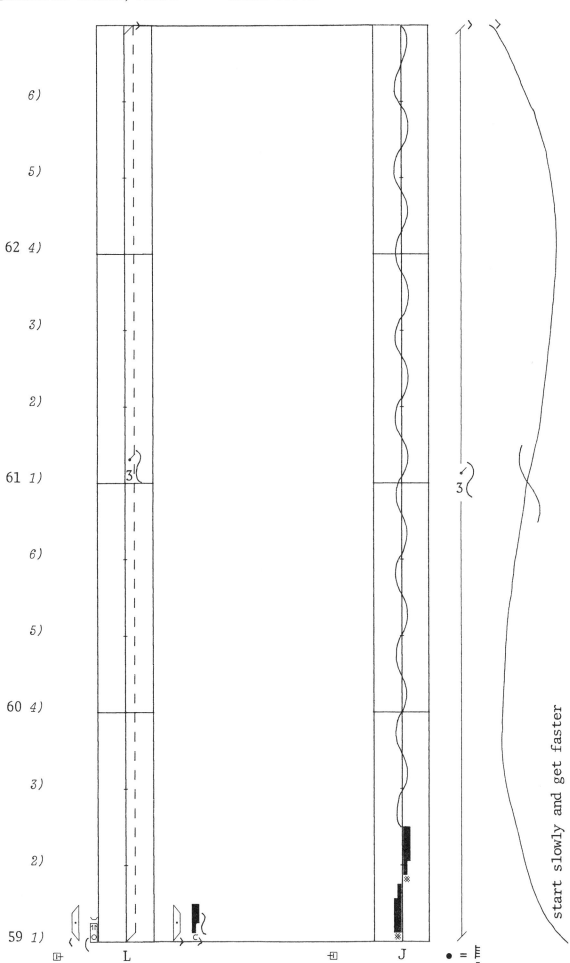

start slowly and get faster

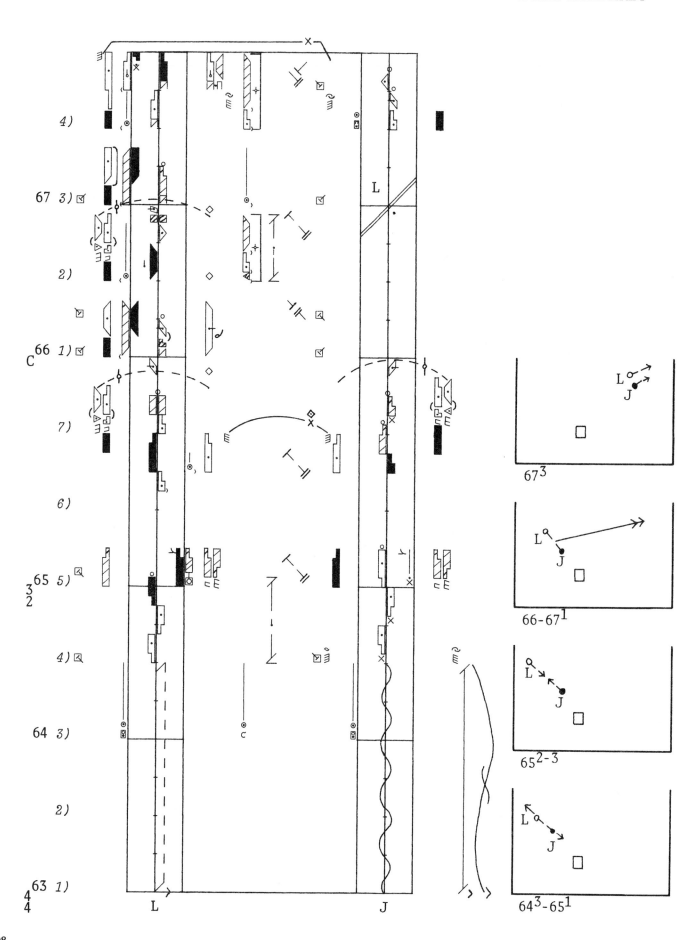

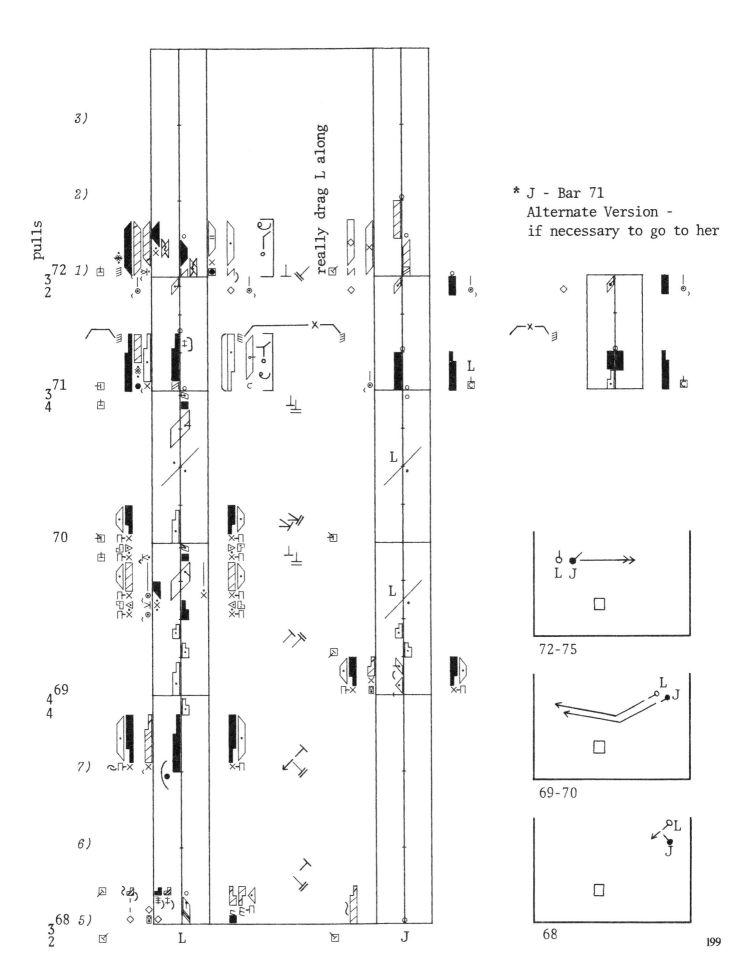

* J - Bar 71
Alternate Version -
if necessary to go to her

72-75

69-70

68

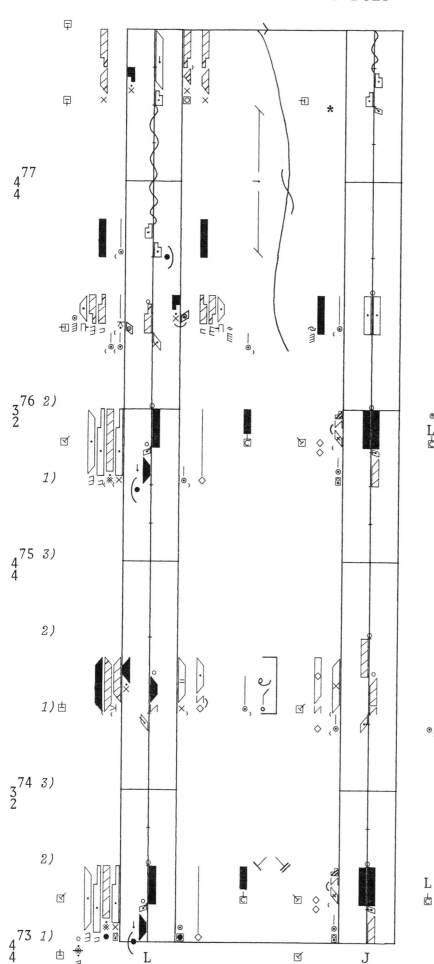

* J - Bar 77²-78
Alternate Version

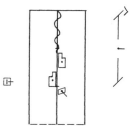

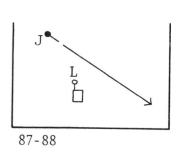

87-88

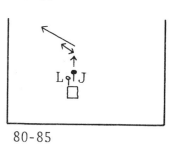

80-85

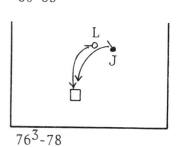

76³-78

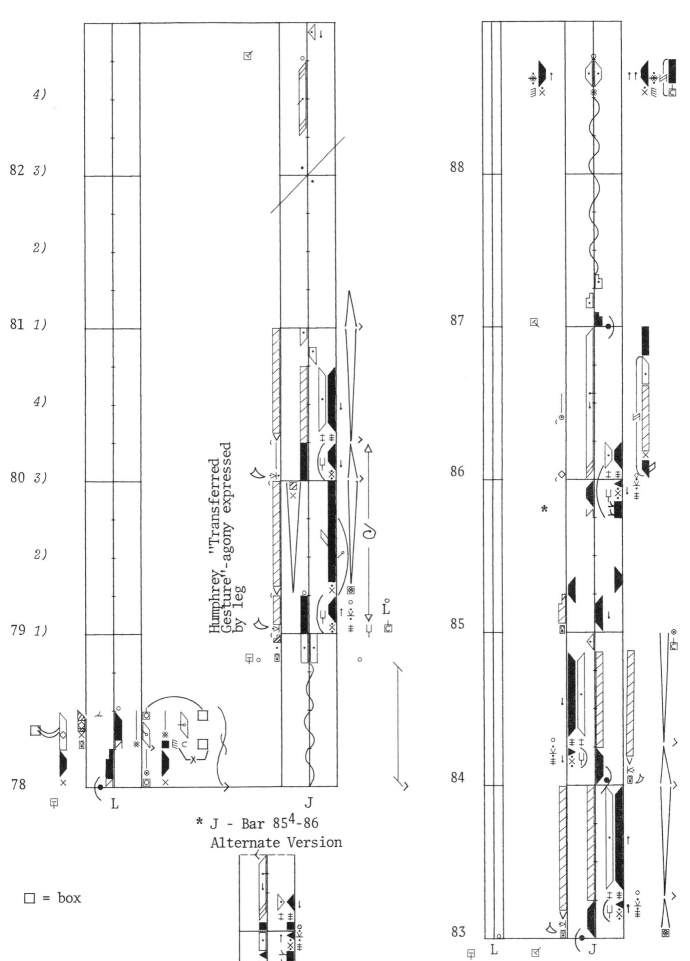

Humphrey, "Transferred Gesture"-agony expressed by leg

* J - Bar 85⁴-86
Alternate Version

□ = box

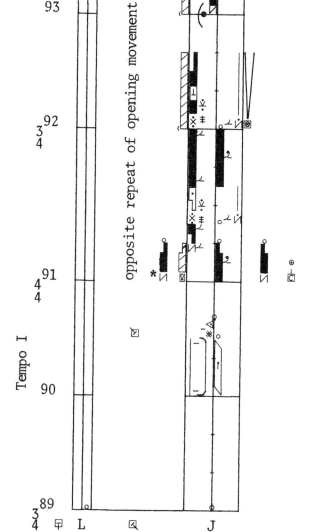

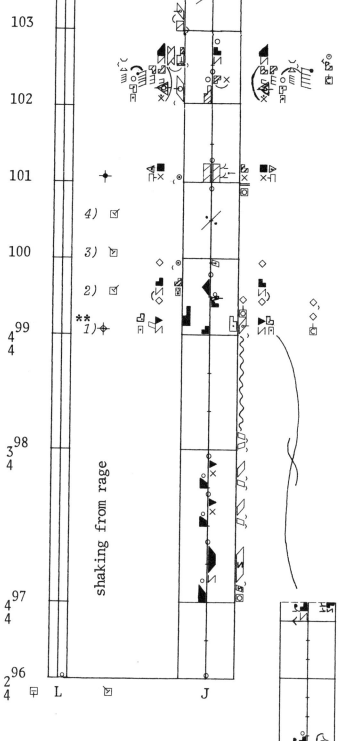

Tempo I

opposite repeat of opening movement

shaking from rage

*J-Bar 91-93[1]

Alternate Version- legs & feet

**♩ = ♪ ; ♪ = ▯

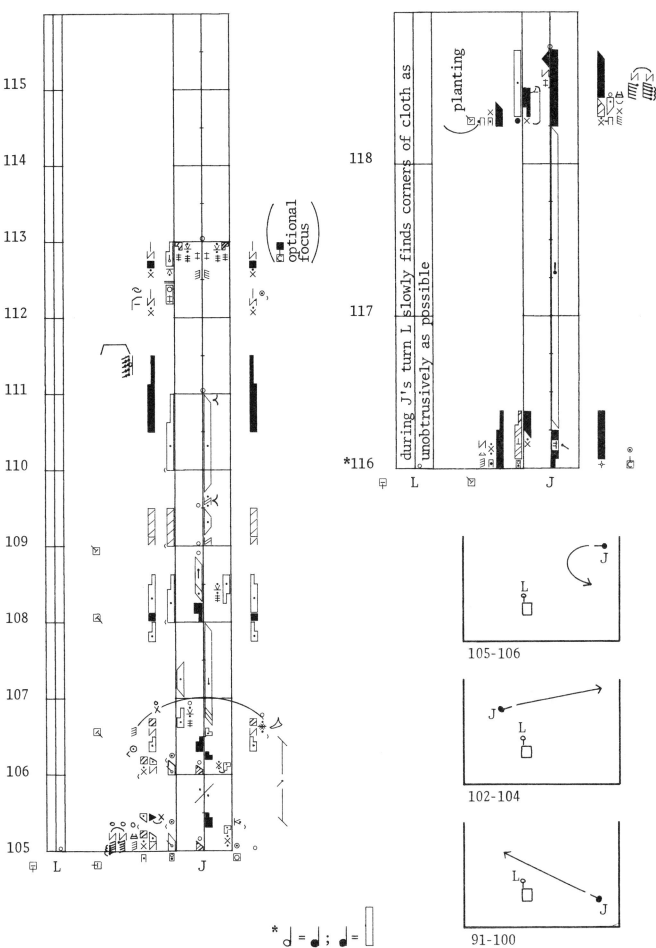

optional focus

planting

during J's turn L slowly finds corners of cloth as unobtrusively as possible

105-106

102-104

91-100

4)

123 3)

2)

$\frac{4}{4}$122 ②

6)

$\frac{3}{4}$121 5)

4)

120 3)

2)

*119 ①

be sure to make folding fluid, blend movements together

L

Cloth

J

fold

as L rises, cloth turns upside down

sometime later, slowly

ad lib pause

  = box

* L - Sometime during J's
previous solo L locates the
◄► edges of the cloth and has
her hands already correctly
placed so she can easily grasp
the ◄► with her fingers.

** Reference to cloth
based on this key:

corners 1,2   corners 3,4
◄■► of cloth
is resting
on floor

fold Cloth

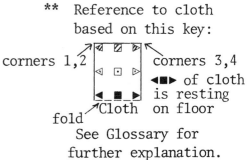

See Glossary for
further explanation.

204

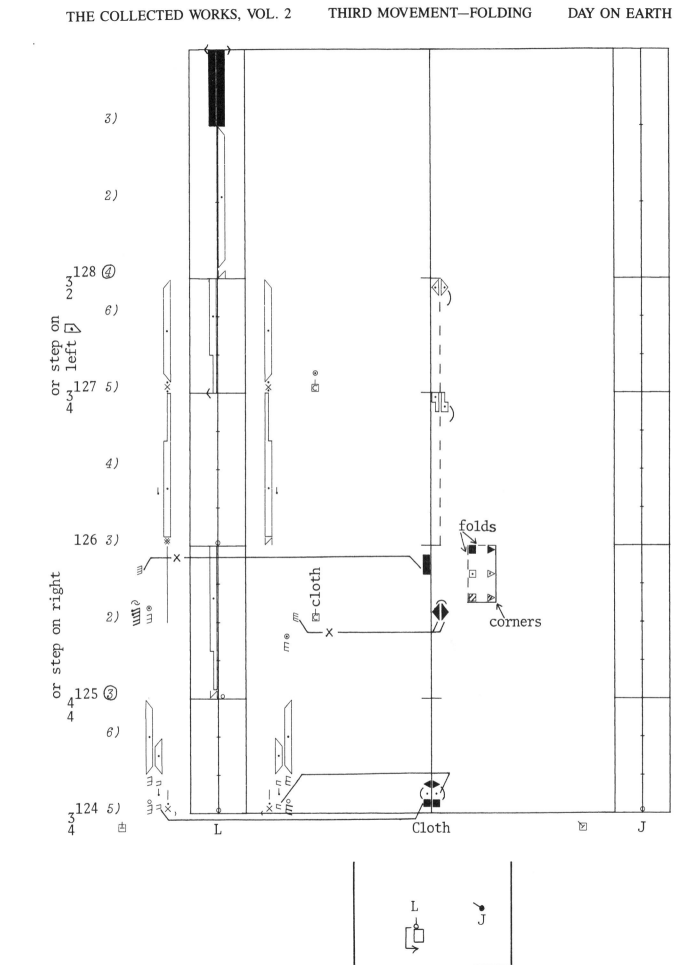

or step on left

or step on right

folds

cloth

corners

L   Cloth   J

L   J

122-128

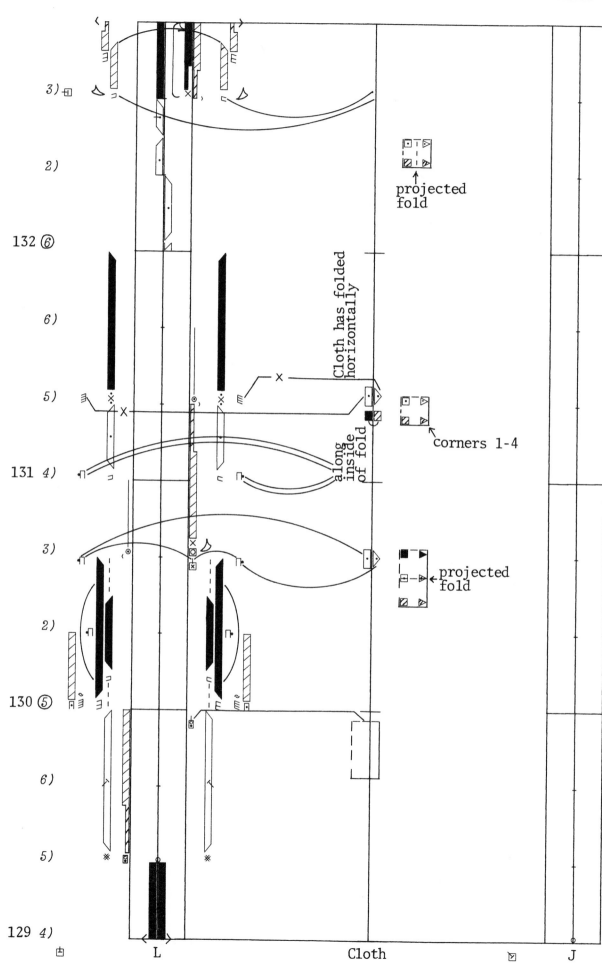

projected
fold

Cloth has folded
horizontally

corners 1-4

along
inside
of fold

projected
fold

3)

2)

132 ⑥

6)

5)

131 4)

3)

2)

130 ⑤

6)

5)

129 4)

L   Cloth   J

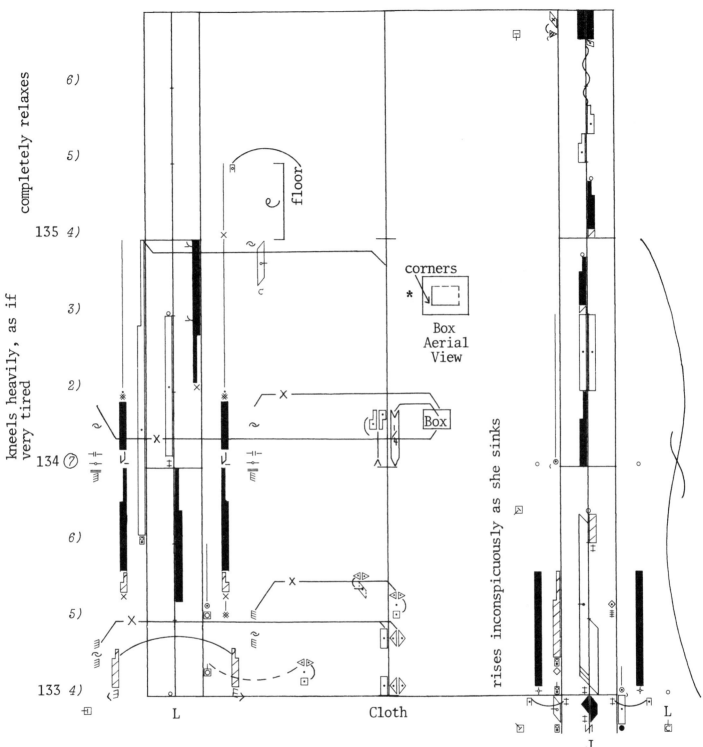

completely relaxes

kneels heavily, as if
very tired

rises inconspicuously as she sinks

floor

corners

*

Box
Aerial
View

Box

6)

5)

135 4)

3)

2)

134 ⑦

6)

5)

133 4)

L

Cloth

J

L

* The cloth must be placed
precisely this way so that
it will unfold properly later.

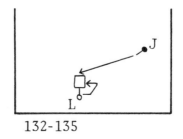

132-135

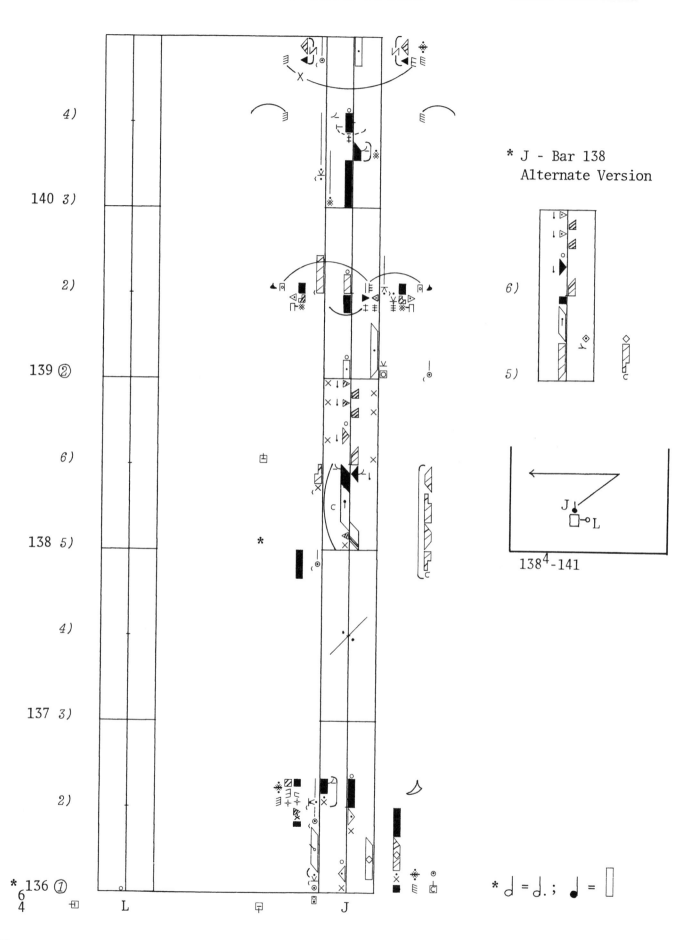

* J - Bar 138
  Alternate Version

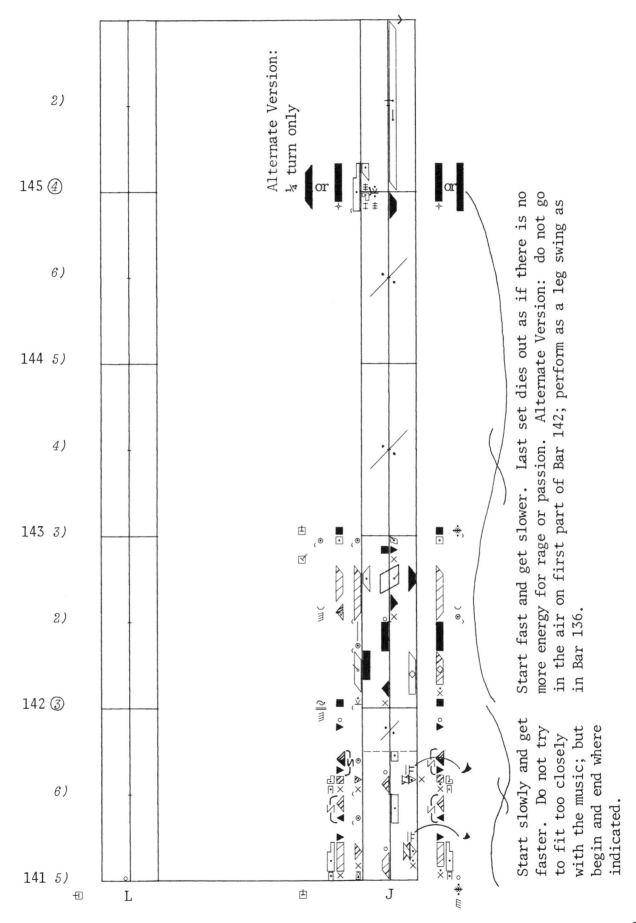

149-152

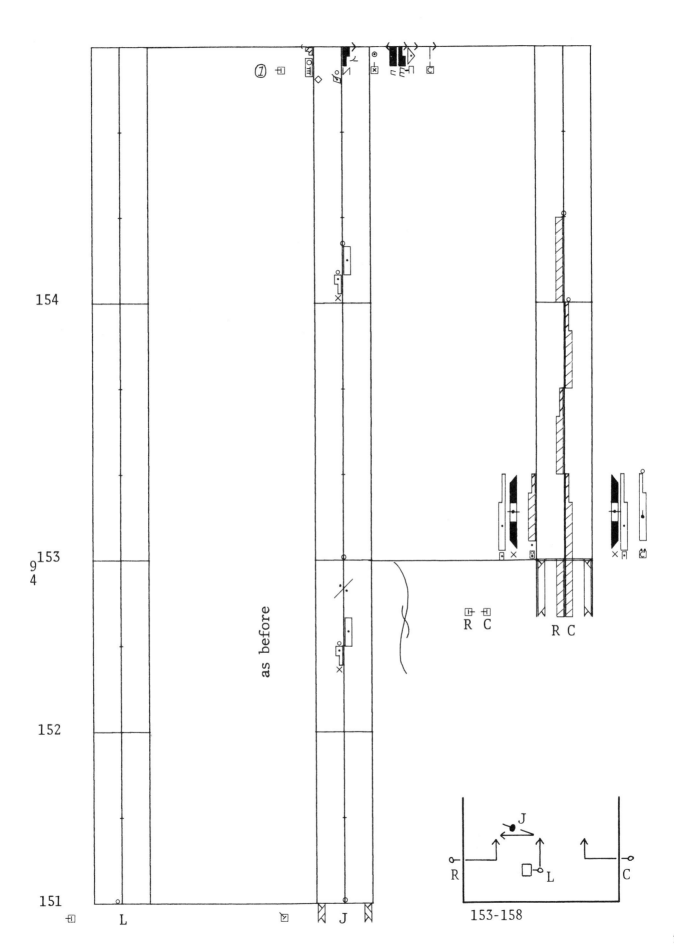

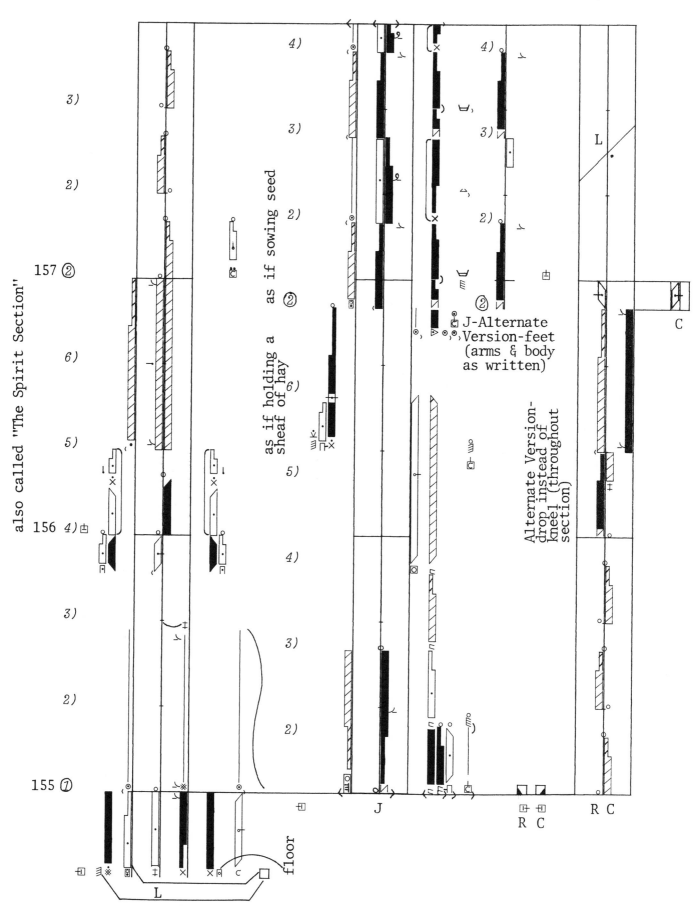

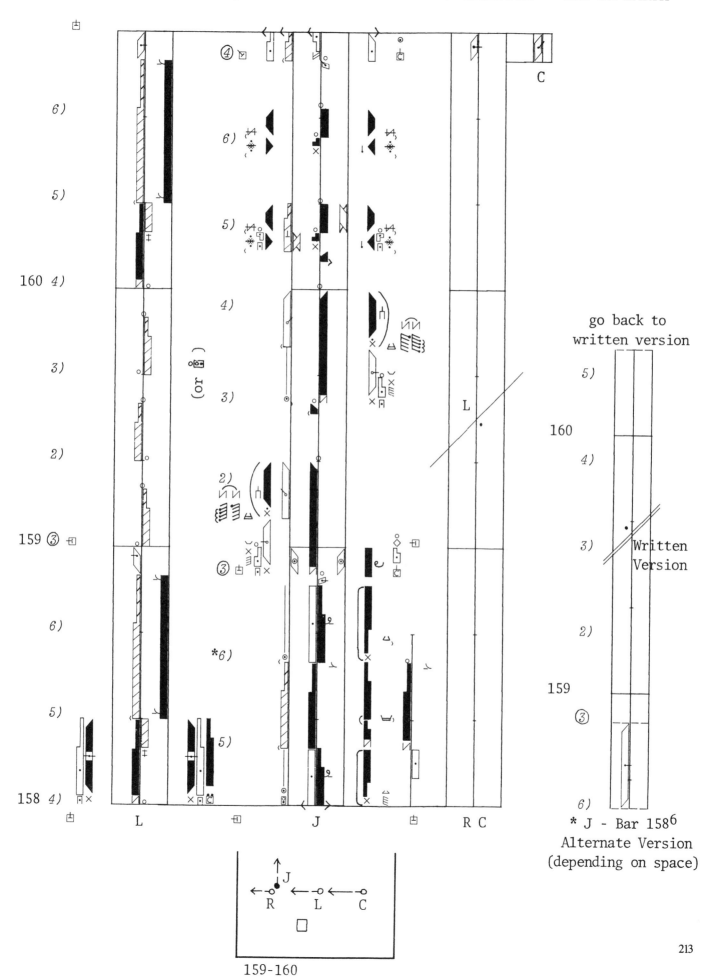

go back to
written version

* J - Bar 158⁶
Alternate Version
(depending on space)

159-160

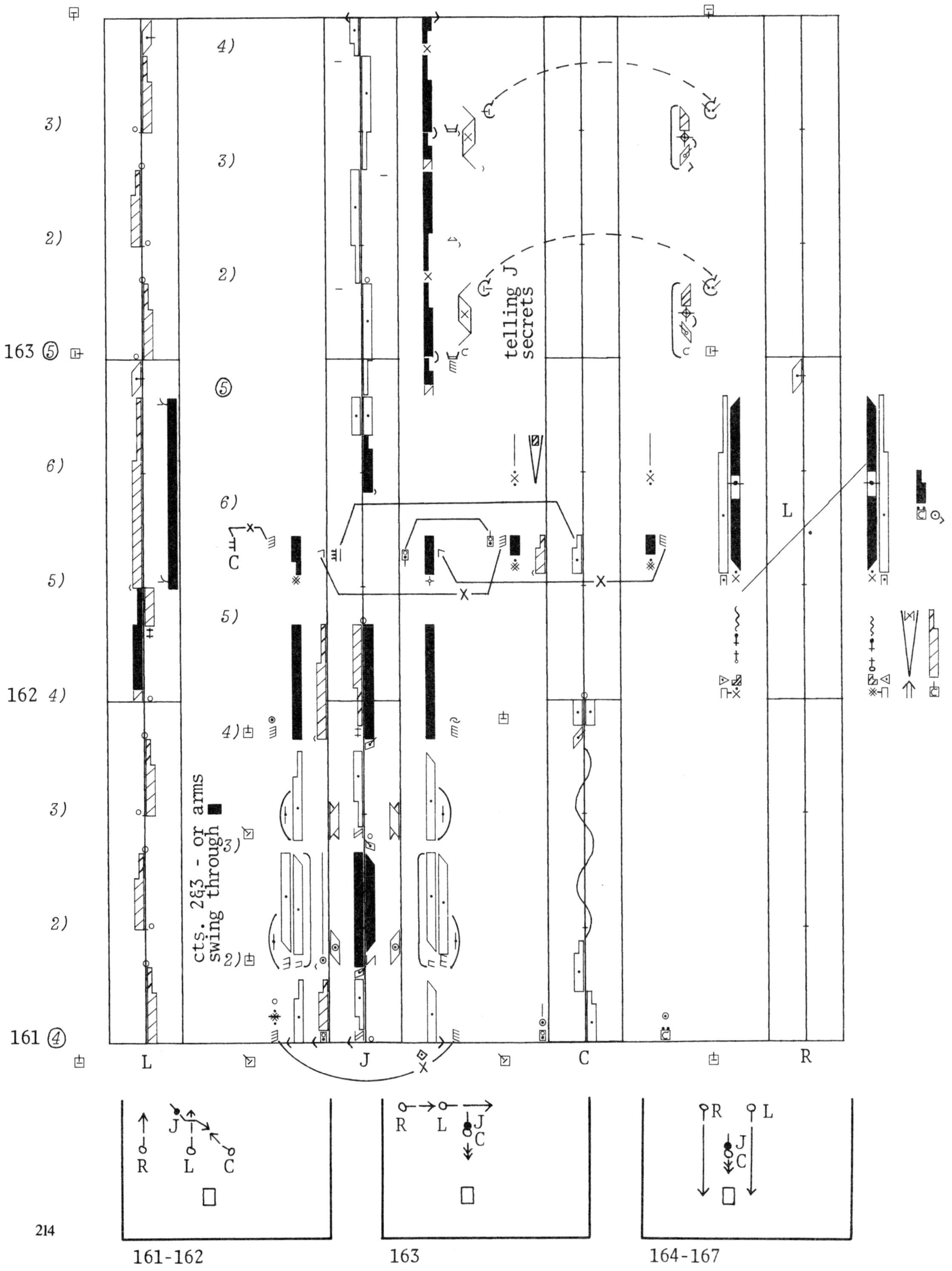

telling J
secrets

cts. 2&3 - or arms
swing through

163 ⑤

162 4)

161 ④

L   J   C   R

161-162   163   164-167

214

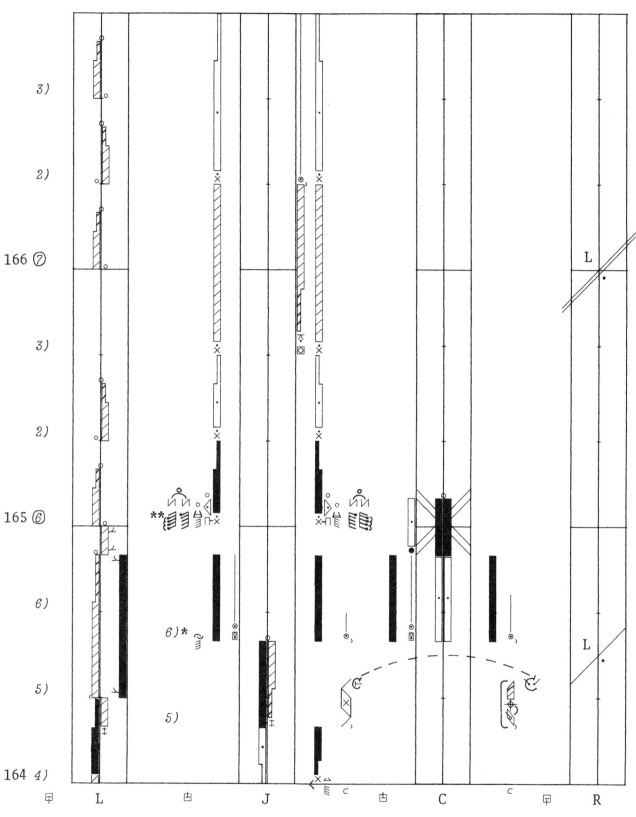

* J - Bar 164[6]
Torso may hold instead
of returning to normal.
It would then go to ▱
on Bar 165[3].

** J - Bar 165
Hands may do this at end of
Bar 166, ct. 1, at the top of
the gesture.

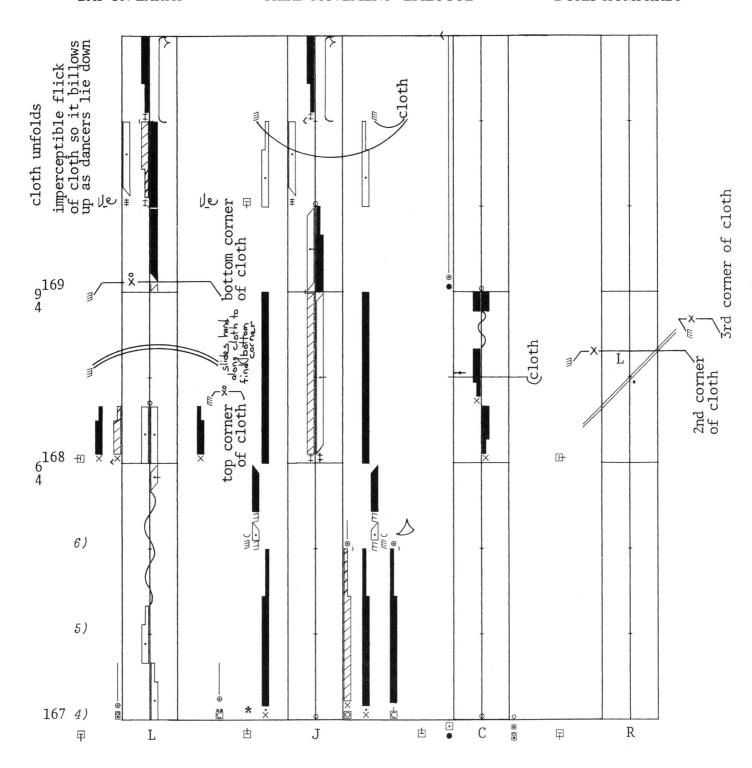

cloth unfolds
imperceptible flick
of cloth so it billows
up as dancers lie down

bottom corner
of cloth

cloth

slides hand
along cloth to
find bottom
corner

top corner
of cloth

cloth

3rd corner of cloth

2nd corner
of cloth

L

9 169
4

6 168
4

6)

5)

167 4)

L   J   C   R

* J - Bar 167
Alternate Version

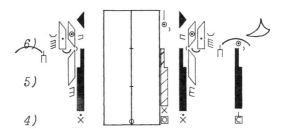

6)

5)

4)

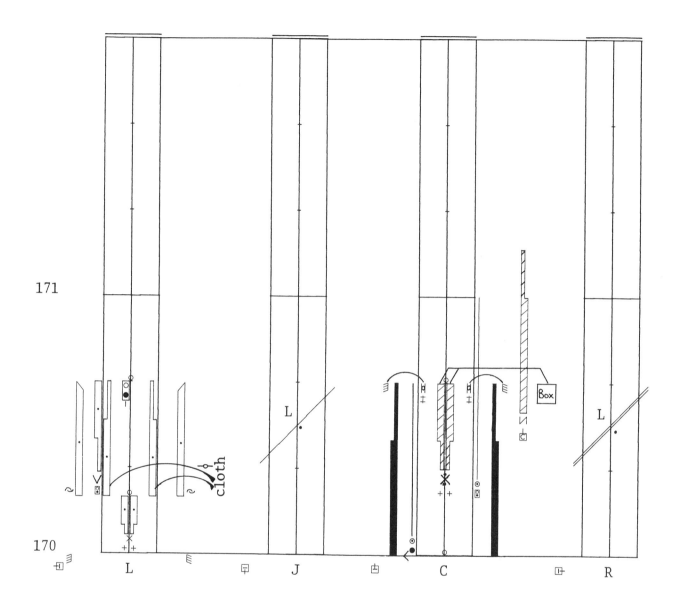

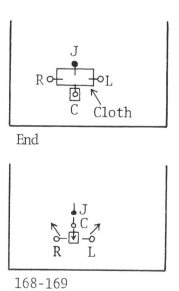

End